To my friend and
now long term
colleague Jim Lieberman!
We both share
a different appreciation
for Tom's ideas. As Fritz
Perls once said, "Good
contact is The appreciation
of differences!" I look forward to
good conversation again
Warmly,

Schaler

Thomas S. Szasz

1920 - 2012
(age 92)

— To Ron Leifer

Homo sum: humani nil a me alienum puto.
("I am a human being: I regard nothing of human
concern as foreign to my interests.")
Terence (Publius Terentius Afer, c. 195/185–c. 159? BC)

Thomas S. Szasz

The Man and His Ideas

Jeffrey A. Schaler
Henry Zvi Lothane
Richard E. Vatz
editors

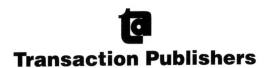

Transaction Publishers

Transaction Publishers is an imprint of the Taylor & Francis Group, an informa business

Library of Congress Cataloging-in-Publication Data: A catalog record for this title has been applied for.
ISBN: 978-1-4128-6514-2
Printed in the United States of America

Contents

Acknowledgments

I acknowledge Tom's early influence on my humanistic and personalistic approach to treating patients in psychotherapy, especially with his book *The Ethics of Psychoanalysis: The Theory and Method of Autonomous Psychotherapy*. On the dust jacket of my book *In Defense of Schreber: Soul Murder and Psychiatry* (1992) he wrote: "a work of monumental and painstaking scholarship by a multilingual polymath and psychoanalyst." The book was reviewed by Rosemary Dinnage in *New York Review of Books* (1994), citing Szasz's ideas.

—HZL

I authored my early book on Szasz with Lee S. Weinberg of the University of Pittsburgh. My numerous conversations and publications on Szasz with Lee have been instrumental to my appreciation of all things Szaszian. In addition I have decades of collegial collaboration with the primary author of this collection, Jeff Schaler. My indebtedness to him cannot be exaggerated. I also owe debts of intellectual growth on Thomas Szasz to my friend Ron Rabin and the man who introduced me to Szaszian work, my greatest professor, graduate or undergraduate, Dr. Trevor Melia. And, of course, years of personal interaction and e-mails with Tom himself were irreplaceable. He has affected every aspect of my academic work.

—REV

I deeply appreciate the thousands of students who loved and challenged me on everything I taught them about Thomas Szasz and his ideas since 1990. I also acknowledge my colleagues at American University in Washington, DC, although some of them in opposition to the seminal precept of academic freedom wanted to—and indeed did—punish professors and students who simply disagreed with psychiatric orthodoxy. As Tom liked to say, "no good deed shall go unpunished." I taught my students to be courageous and autonomous and I always warned them that freedom of speech is never free. A special thank you to the wonderful contributors to this book for trusting me. Indeed, I should like to express a special note of appreciation to Rick Vatz, my good friend and colleague for collaborating and guiding me over many years, as we both dealt with the fall-out from our controversial writings published in the court of public opinion, as well as through the treacherous waters of academia. Thank you for coming on board as co-editor, Rick, especially when I was left high and dry; and finally to Dr. David Ramsay Steele, another close friend of mine for many years, and personal editor, who continues to "save me from myself."

I dedicate this book and my intellectual and academic life work to my wonderful daughter Magda. As Tom said to me at your wedding, Magda, tongue-in-cheek, grinning, in his thick Hungarian accent, "Jeff! . . . You certainly did something right!"

I remember when the three of us were walking to HBO studios in Manhattan for the first of many televised debates and Tom said to you, "Magda, needless to say, your father is very proud of you!" I am proud of you, Magda, and I will always love you.

—JAS

Introduction

Henry Zvi Lothane

Instead of producing a run of the mill introduction offering insipid summaries of the ideas discussed in this volume, which the reader can find easily by reading the actual chapters, I feel impelled to offer a reflection on the man and his work stemming from some parallels in our itineraries. Before coming to America we were first raised and educated in central Europe, he in Hungary me in Poland. We were both refugees from Hitler: he went west coming to the United States from France; I went east, first to Russia then back to Poland, and after years in Israel to the United States. Early on we were both interested in literature and philosophy and even though we graduated from medical schools, we forsook the career of a "real" doctor practicing internal medicine and became psychiatrists and psychoanalysts. When I started my residency in psychiatry in Rochester, New York, in 1963 I had the good fortune of becoming acquainted with two Hungarian psychoanalysts: first with Sandor Feldman in Rochester and then with Thomas Szasz in Syracuse. These men became role models and inspired me to become an analyst. It is with Tom that I developed a dialogue and a friendship that lasted for years until his death, exchanging ideas and citing each other's works. Sandor Feldman taught me to seek truth and confront falsehood in communicating with the other, Thomas Szasz—the ethics of defending patients' civil liberties, which I pursued in my 1992 book *In Defense of Schreber*, a victim of psychiatric incarceration at the turn of the twentieth century, and in my practice of psychotherapy. The idea of freedom was further implemented by Szasz to promote the concept of autonomous psychotherapy (Szasz, 1962).

In his 2004 "Autobiographical Sketch," Szasz describes how he "realized, even before [he] left Hungary, that psychiatry and psychoanalysis had nothing to do with real medicine or with one another: psychiatrists locked up troublesome persons in insane asylums" (Schaler, 2004, pp. 17–18). What he omitted mentioning were his roots in and identification with the tradition of Hungarian freedom fighters, such as Lajos Kossuth, a peerless orator, patriot statesman and exile, and the appeal of the land of the free and of free speech. The shocking title "Myth of Mental Illness" was not a scheme to destroy psychiatry but a freedom manifesto of a self-proclaimed second Pinel, a battle cry to restore dignity and freedom of choice to asylum inmates, a serious call to becoming a critic of the psychiatric profession and urging it to examine its ethics and procedures. It was a voice of conscience that every profession needs. And institutional psychiatry of the 1960s was still closer to the conditions described in Felix Deutsch's exposé *The Shame of the States* in the 1940s than to the psychiatry we practice today, for which credit is due to Thomas Szasz's long-lasting crusade and the dismantling of the old mammoth asylums like Pilgrim State Hospital initiated by the New York State Office of Mental Health in Albany. With the spread of community psychiatry, imported from England, former inmates were transferred to residential treatment centers.

These were also the times of growing public awareness of the need for humane reforms of the psychiatric hospital system as epitomized in Ken Kesey's 1962 novel *One Flew Over the Cuckoo's Nest*, first adapted into a Broadway play and then into a film by Miklos Forman, to win five Academy Awards. Instead of being recognized, Szasz was repeatedly crucified as a renegade, a stormy petrel, if not plain psychotic, trials which he both endured and relished. This tragic misunderstanding makes me see him as a tragic figure.

Szasz's other message of *The Myth of Mental Illness*, actually the more important philosophical legacy, was promoting *interpersonal* psychiatry and psychoanalysis with an emphasis on communication and dialogue; on roles, rules, and relations; and on games people play; and last and not least, on psychiatry and the law. Accordingly, he cited the many ideas of many predecessors in this venture: Jurgen Ruesch and Gregory Bateson, Harry Stack Sullivan, Jean Piaget, Eric Berne as well as philosophers such as John Dewey, George Herbert Meade, and Bertrand Russell. In this connection it is helpful to quote from Szasz's 1961 "The use of names and the origin of the myth of mental illness," published before the book came out (*American*

Psychologist, 16(2):59–65). In this paper, Szasz addressed the triple function of language:

> to transmit information, to induce mood, and to promote action. . . . Since the social sciences, psychiatry among them, are concerned . . . with how people influence each other—the so-called promotive use of language is a significant part of the observational data they endeavor to describe and explain. A major source of difficulty in such undertakings is that the social sciences themselves use everyday language which is often logically obscure or ambiguous which lends itself readily to promotive rather than cognitive usage. (p. 59)

Szasz did not tire of emphasizing that the way we speak determines the way we act. And I might add: not just everyday language, scientific language, is beset by the same dilemma as well: it often conceals promotive messages under the guise of cognitive assertions. Whether such cognitive assertions are valid may be a problem, too, but that is a task for another day.

Like many other refugees from dictatorships and unfreedom, Szasz not only fell under the spell of the American promise of life, liberty, and the pursuit of happiness but became a libertarian fighting for the liberties of freedom-deprived asylum inmates. For this he reaped both recognition and rejection. The latter may have tinged his life with some disappointment, if not unhappiness, but it never led to despair. Arriving in America without speaking a word of English Szasz became a consummate master of the language both as speaker and writer, let alone brilliant aphorist in the style of Friedrich Nietzsche and Oscar Wilde. Here is an example: "Freedom is what most people want for themselves, and what they most want to deprive others of" (Szasz, 1973).

References

Schaler, J. A. (Ed.). (2004). *Szasz under fire the psychiatric abolitionist faces his critics.* Chicago, IL and La Salle, IL: Open Court.

Szasz, T. (1962). Human nature and psychotherapy: A further contribution to the theory of autonomous psychotherapy. *Comprehensive Psychiatry, 3*(5), 268–283.

Szasz, T. (1974). *The Second Sin* (p. 41). New York: Anchor Press.

Part I

Psychiatry and the World after Szasz

1

Reminiscences of Thomas Szasz and His Ideas

Henry Zvi Lothane

After three decades of friendship with Szasz—born on April 15, 1920, died on September 8, 2012—I eulogized him in the obituary the *Times* (London) invited me to write. Immediately below is what I submitted:

> Thomas Szasz, doctor of medicine, emeritus Professor of Psychiatry at SUNY, Syracuse, psychoanalyst and member of the International and American Psychoanalytic Associations, died after a fall at age 92, ending a long publishing career from 1947 to 2011. He became the best known and the most controversial psychiatrist in America and beyond following the publication of his 1961 book, *The Myth of Mental Illness*, subtitled *Foundations of a Theory of Personal Conduct*. Supported by a only a handful but branded in overwhelming numbers of his psychiatric colleagues as a denigrator, a fouler of his own nest, provocateur and traitor, let alone a paranoid schizophrenic, Szasz ignited highly emotional and acrimonious wars of words that are still continuing. In 2004, his follower, psychologist Jeffrey A. Schaler, edited *Szasz Under Fire: The Psychiatric Abolitionist Faces his Critics*, with Szasz's own autobiographical sketch and responses to his critics (the quotes and material below are from that book).

> *1920*

> Thomas Stephen Szasz was the second son born in Budapest to the upper middle class housewife Lily and Julius Szász, a businessman. They were assimilated Jews who celebrated Christmas. He loved his mother and respected his father. He was a sickly child and nearly died of diphtheria: "My illnesses taught me the advantages of being ill: I knew what 'secondary gain' was decades before I heard the term and I learned to malinger." He emigrated to the USA in 1938 and started his medical studies in 1941, completing a medical residency and subsequently a psychiatric residency. By 1950 he graduated from

3

the Chicago Psychoanalytic Institute whose director was another Hungarian emigré, Franz Alexander, a leader in psychoanalysis and psychosomatic medicine. In 1951 he became a board certified psychiatrist.

Szasz argued that whereas medicine dealt with real illness of diseased organs, psychiatry was concerned with a mythical, that is, meta-phorical, both fictitious and factitious, illness, a kind of malingering. However, he did not deny that "problems of living" are real but that such problems are part of psychology and sociology and have their legal, economic, social, and political aspects. Lost in the shuffle was the influence upon Szasz of a great American psychiatrist, Harry Stack Sullivan, who also portrayed psychiatric disorders as a problem in living, propounding a psychological and sociological conception of schizophrenia.

These views led Szasz to decry psychiatric diagnoses as fiction and to advance "a body of pleading of replacing psychiatric control and coercion with psychiatric cooperation and contract" and in 1970, together with sociologist Erving Goffman and lawyer George J. Alexander, to found the American Association for the Abolition of Involuntary Mental Hospitalization and its journal, *The Abolitionist*, campaigning that "both civil commitment and the insanity defense should be abolished." Such a program and the rhetoric of "comparing psychiatric patients with slaves and psychiatrists with slaveholders" exacerbated the polarization even more. What was lost in these polemics was Szasz's positive libertarian message: his humanism, his concern for the rights of the individual vs. the state, big business, or any other collectivist interest, criticized in his writings as "pharmac-racy" and "the therapeutic state." Let us not forget: Szasz may have also been reacting not only to the Holocaust but to the enslavement of his native Hungary by the Russian dictators. Not only was Szasz a staunch freedom fighter, he was tenacious in his responses to oppo-nents. One is reminded of George Bernard Shaw's condemnation of vaccination or Oscar Wilde's epigrams.

However, two issues beg the question in this debate. If psychiatry, as he claimed, was a metaphorical profession treating a metaphorical illness, the same could be said of medicine: in overwhelming numbers, patients who visit doctors or hospital emergency rooms complain of various sensations that are *not* caused by lesions in organs but are bodily metaphors of emotional experiences and cries for help addressed to the doctor. From 1947 to 1957, still under the influence of the psychosomatics of Franz Alexander, Szasz published on the psychosomatic connection between feelings and the body, for exam-ple, "The psychology of bodily feelings in schizophrenia," or the book *Pain and Pleasure: A Study of Bodily Feelings*. Thus, depending on the person and the life situation, body and mind may function as a metaphor for each other.

The other questions concern the role of coercion in society. For example, a person may not shout fire in a theatre filled with people and claim the First Amendment. Such an act may either be seen as a felony punishable by law with imprisonment or as folly justifying involuntary psychiatric hospitalization. Either way, society needs to control antisocial behavior whether it be labeled as immoral or illegal, sinful or sick. While Szasz seems to favor the 'honest' legal control over the 'hypocritical' psychiatric control, his main impact and intention should be seen as a crusade similar to Freud's at the turn of the 20th century: to humanize the psychiatric profession, to make it interpersonal, to institute checks and balances against the temptation to become autocratic and despotic, as happened so many times to so many psychiatrists and their patients. For this Szasz deserves our everlasting gratitude. Szasz's ethical message still rings true today as psychiatry, or healing the soul with empathy and sympathy is tempted to go scientific and regulate the brain with drugs. It is not a matter of an either/or but seeking an integrative approach to healing the whole person which requires regulating body and mind.

I met Szasz in 1964 and we became friends. In all those years he was a genteel interlocutor and wise guide.

Szasz's former wife Rosine committed suicide in 1971, following their divorce. He is survived by daughters Dr. Margot Szasz Peters and Suzy Szasz Palmer, and one grandson, Andrew Peters. His brother George died soon after Szasz's own death. The two were very close.

The *Times'* obituary editors not only shortened and substantially edited what I submitted, but also failed to identify me as the author! The obituary was published anonymously in the *Times* on October 11, 2012: "Dr. Thomas Szasz psychiatrist and psychoanalyst who challenged the medical world with deeply unconventional views on the nature of mental illness" (p. 54).

When First Szasz and I Met

Szasz and I met in 1964 when he was a Professor of Psychiatry at Syracuse University's Department of Psychiatry, chaired by Marc Hollender, MD., and I, a resident in psychiatry at Strong Memorial Hospital in Rochester, New York and the Rochester University Department of Psychiatry, founded by Distinguished Professor and Chairman Dr. John Romano, who was not an analyst, even though in the 1940s he had been a fellow in psychoanalysis in Boston together with Charles Brenner.

Some Personal Memories

Here are the events that led to my encounter with Szasz. After graduating as an MD from the Hebrew University Hadassah Medical School in Jerusalem in 1960, during my subsequent internship at Beilinson Hospital, I met Dr. Roy Waldman from Long Beach, NY and we became friends. He suggested I take the American foreign graduate examination (ECFMG) in case I would decide one day to study psychiatry in the United States. It happened sooner than I imagined. I took the exam and applied to a number of Eastern residency training programs. While awaiting the decision I spent nine months as resident in psychiatry at the Talbieh Psychiatric Hospital in Jerusalem led by Professor Heinrich Winnick, noted psychiatrist and psychoanalyst. I recall him saying that in America, to be somebody in psychiatry you had to be an analyst. At Talbieh I worked in a closed female ward, did not attend any courses, and scored some successes treating my women patients with common sense and empathy which my chief attributed to beginners' luck.

Before settling down in Rochester I spent some days with the Waldmans in Syracuse, where Roy was already a politically active second year resident in psychiatry (see Schaler, 2004, p. 395). I continued to visit Roy who introduced me to Szasz's ideas. One day I attended a teaching session led by Szasz and met him in person and in time the encounter blossomed into a friendship.

Meeting Szasz in Syracuse was a mind-blowing experience for me, compared with the traditional psychiatric atmosphere in Rochester. Older Rochester psychiatrists and analysts seemed to espouse ideas similar to Szasz, for example, Chicago trained Gordon Pleune (1965). Despite John Romano's distancing himself from psychoanalysis after a sabbatical in England, psychoanalytic teaching was still strong in the Department even as it was now veering toward community psychiatry and actuarial research. Faculty members pursuing analytic training were analyzed by one of the two analysts in town, Sandor Feldman or Sidney Rubin, and shuttled on weekends to the Downstate Institute in Brooklyn to attend courses.

Another wonderful teacher was George L. Engel, a physician but not a psychiatrist, who was also trained in Chicago. He was a master at interviewing medical patients with a free-associative technique first described by Felix Deutsch. Engel's likening the so-called hysteric's behavior to the game of charades was in keeping with Szasz's game theory analysis of such conduct but there was no love lost between them (see the remark by Szasz about Engel in Schaler, p. 49). Otherwise, starting with John Romano down, everybody was hostile to and suspicious of Szasz's ideas about psychiatry. Thus one of the chief residents, Dr. Frederick Glaser (1965), acted as mouthpiece of this opposition discussing Szasz's 1963 book *Law, Liberty, and Psychiatry*:

> The dialectic of law and psychiatry is hardly a closed issue, and certain of Dr. Szasz's points will have to be taken into account, at least, if a more satisfactory synthesis is to be achieved. One of the saddening aspects of his present book is that, because its strident tone, the baby may be lost in the bathwater. Many may, in their reaction to the excremental vision of American psychiatry, completely discount everything he has to say. . . . The question will inevitably be raised whether sanctions of some form ought to be taken against Dr. Szasz, not only because of the content of his views but because of the manner in which he presents them. He has not chosen to limit his discussion to professional circles, as his magazine article (not the first that he has written) testifies. In fact, he announces in the preface of his book that such dissemination is a part of his program, in a manner which seems to enjoin the raising of the standard of revolt (i–viii): "the book is addressed not only to lawyers, psychiatrists, and social scientists but also to intelligent laymen. Indeed the last may find it especially useful, for organized psychiatry poses a much graver threat to him than it does to the professionals." Certain it is that Dr. Szasz's writings will have devastating effects. (p. 1073)

I am not aware that such stones were ever thrown at any other American critic of psychiatry. Canadian-American sociologist Erving Goffman (not mentioned by Glaser) published his most famous book *Asylums* in 1961, the same year as Szasz's *The Myth of Mental Illness*. Also influential, in Europe, more than in the United States, were the 1961 Michel Foucault's *Folie et deraison. Histoire de la folie a l'age classique* (*madness and civilization in the age of reason*) and the 1969 Klaus Dörner's *Bürger und Irre Zur Sozialgeschichte und Wissenschaftssoziologie der Psychiatrie* (*madman and bourgeois: A social science oriented history of psychiatry*). Goffman tellingly characterized the asylums as a "total institutions" of which there were "five groupings":

> [1] Institutions established to care for persons felt to be incapable and harmless, these are the homes for the blind; [2] to care for persons felt to be incapable . . . and a threat to the community, albeit an unintended one . . . TB sanitaria, mental hospitals, and leprosaria; [3] organized to protect the community against what are felt to be intentional dangers

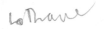

to it: jails, penitentiaries, P.O.W. camps, and concentration camps; [4] institutions [for] for some worklike task . . . : army barracks, ships, boarding schools, work camps . . . ; [5] retreats from the world . . . : abbeys, monasteries, convents, and other cloisters . . . a classification not neat or exhaustive. (pp. 4–5)

Szasz's use of the word myth produced seismic shocks but did not devastate psychiatry. And we shouldn't fault Szasz for having used a provocative title to call attention to his ideas seeing how he imitated Freud having shocked his Viennese colleagues presenting cases of *male* hysteria or calling an infant's sucking at the breast sexual. Concerning myths, Freud wrote in 1933 responding to Einstein: "It may perhaps seem to you as though our theories are a kind of mythology and, in the present case, not even an agreeable one. But does not every science come in the end to a kind of mythology like this? Cannot the same be said to-day of your own Physics?" (p. 211).

My decision to apply for analytic training in New York during my residency had multiple inspirations: teachers like Dan Schuster, Otto Thaler, and Sidney Rubin, and above all Sandor Feldman, like Szasz, another naturalized son of Hungarian Jews from Budapest, who once a week at 9:00 p.m. came from his home to teach a small self-selected group of residents: he read to us his notes of a three-year long analysis of a woman and kept adding new cases and examples to his fascinating book on mannerisms of speech and gestures in everyday life (Feldman, 1959).

But I was also influenced by Szasz. In all those years Szasz was for me a genteel interlocutor and wise guide. He wrote a great blurb for my 1992 book on Schreber and cited me in a number of his later books for which I in turn reciprocated with citing him and with blurbs for his books. A book that influenced my work with patients was his 1965 *The Ethics of Psychoanalysis*, in which he made reference to his *Myth of Mental Illness*.

Szasz's Ideas on Freedom

Freedom and choice, as manifestations of autonomy and free will and an opposite of hard or soft determinism, are not usually discussed by psychiatrists or psychoanalysts. Approaching "the problem of freedom" in 1965 Szasz defined the meaning of "psychiatric symptoms" as "ideas, feelings, inclinations and *actions* that are considered undesirable, involuntary, or alien [thus] inappropriate [as judged by] the client himself; his relatives; the expert sympathetic with his desires; an expert openly or covertly antagonistic to him; or, finally by society in general . . . All entail an essential restriction of the patient's freedom to engage in conduct available to others similarly situated in society . . . The common element in these and other so-called psychiatric symptoms is the expression of loss of control or freedom" (p. 13–14; emphasis added).

Applying the idea of freedom to psychotherapy, Szasz noted that "Freud's great contribution lies in having laid the foundation for a therapy that seeks to enlarge the patient's choices and hence his freedom and responsibility" (p. 16). Note that the man who called mental illness a myth did not shy from calling the client a patient and continues: "Since Freud's death, the aim of analysis has been to free the patient from the constricting effects of his neurosis (the term neurosis meaning unconsciously determined, stereotyped behavior, in contrast to 'normal,' freely chosen, consciously determined conduct) . . . to give patients constrained by their habitual patterns of action greater freedom in their personal conduct . . . defined in terms of goals that man must establish for himself. This is the kind of freedom that no one can give another" (pp. 17–19).

Szasz and Essentialism versus Operationalism

Interestingly, the word myth was not in the index of Szasz's 1965 book while the words freedom and liberty were not indexed in the 1961 book, nor was myth defined in an article entitled "the myth of mental illness" Szasz published in 1960, where he stated:

> While I have argued that mental illnesses do not exist, I obviously did not imply that the social and psychological occurrences to which this *label* is currently being attached also do not exist. Like the personal and social troubles which people had in the Middle Ages, they are real enough. *It is the labels we give them that concerns us and, having labeled them, what we do about them.* While I cannot go into the ramified implications of this problem herein, it is worth noting that a demonologic conception of problems in living gave rise to therapy along theological lines. Today, a belief in mental illness implies—nay, requires—therapy along medical or psychotherapeutic lines. (p. 117; emphasis added)

A label is literally, a slip, for example, of paper inscribed and affixed to something for identification or description, or figuratively, a descriptive or identifying word, phrase, or epithet. While acknowledging that social troubles were real, Szasz suggested it is the label that is unreal but he did not suggest a better label or name. But mark well: Szasz questioned the reality of an imprecise term, without any mention of disorder or diagnosis, but at the same time amenable to therapy along medical or psychotherapeutic lines, thus pitting the unreality of the label against the reality of the treatment, an inconsistency in his argument. Finally, the word mental per se was not questioned, only the word disease; but while in the standard dictionaries "disease" and "illness" are both defined literally as referring to diseased organs and figuratively to a disturbed mind, Szasz focused on the literal meaning only. Szasz concluded as follows:

> I have tried to show that the notion of mental illness has outlived whatever usefulness it might have had and that it now functions merely as a convenient myth. As such, *it is a true heir to religious myths in general,* and to the belief in witchcraft in particular; the role of all these belief systems was to act as *social tranquilizers,* thus encouraging the hope that mastery of certain specific problems may be achieved by means of substitutive (symbolic-magical) operations. The notion of mental illness thus serves mainly to obscure the every-day fact that life for most people is a continuous struggle, not for biological survival, but for a "place in the sun," "peace of mind," or some other human value. For man aware of himself and of the world about him, once the needs for preserving the body (and perhaps the race) are more or less satisfied, the problem arises as to what he should do himself. Sustained adherence to the myth of mental illness allows people to avoid facing this problem, believing that mental health, conceived as the absence of mental illness, automatically insures the making of right and safe choices in one's conduct of life. But the facts are all the other way, it is the making of good choices in life that others regard, retrospectively, as good mental health. The myth of mental illness encourages us, moreover, to believe in its logical corollary: that social intercourse should be harmonious, satisfying, and the secure basis of a "good life" were it not for the disrupting influence of mental illness or "psychopathology." (p. 118; first emphasis added)

The transition from label to myth is abrupt and myth is also left undefined, perhaps because its meaning as a widely held but false belief or idea is so well known. In keeping with the previous passage, the idea that myths and labels are fictions is buttressed by a tantalizing comparison of the notion of mental illness to medieval belief in witchcraft and the word's association of innocent women labeled as witches and tortured to death by the Inquisition. Not surprisingly, this analysis demonstrates the problematic nature of *both* labels, that of mental illness as much as mental health, or the answer to the question "what is a good life?" versus what it "should be." Also, Szasz did not explain how a modern psychological myth is similar to a medieval theological or theology like psychology.

My view of Szasz's medieval analogy, whether he knew it or not, alludes to a philosophical debate that engrossed the minds in the Middle Ages: between realists, like St. Anselm, who believed in the reality of universals, that is, abstract ideas, versus nominalists, like Abelard and William of Ockham, who argued that there are only particulars. As to universals versus particulars in psychiatry and psychoanalysis, both share the use of abstraction and generalization with medicine, as pointed out by physician and Rockefeller University researcher and naturalized Frenchman Alexis Carrel (1935) and which is still true today despite the amazing advances in medical and scientific technology:

> A disease is not an entity. We observe individuals suffering from pneumonia, syphilis, diabetes, typhoid fever, etc. However, it would have been impossible to build up a science of medicine merely by compiling a great number of individual observations. The facts had to be classified and simplified with the aid of abstractions. In this way disease was born. And medical treatises could be written. A kind of science was built up, roughly descriptive, rudimentary, imperfect, but convenient, indefinitely perfectible and easy to teach. Unfortunately, we have been content with this result. We did not understand that treatises describing pathological entities contain only a part of the knowledge indispensable to those who attend to the sick. Medical knowledge should go beyond the science of diseases. The physician must clearly distinguish the sick human being described in his books from the concrete patient whom he has to treat, who must not only be studied, but, above all, relieved, encouraged, and cured. His role is to discover the characteristics of the sick man's individuality . . . [and] the psychological personality of the individual. In fact, medicine which confines itself to the study of diseases, amputates a part of its own body.

> Today the old quarrel of the realists and the nominalists is being revived around the schools of medicine. Scientific medicine, installed in its palaces, defends, as did the church of the Middle Ages, the reality of the Universals. It anathematizes the nominalists, who, following the example of Abelard, consider Universals and disease as creations of our mind, and the patient as the only reality. In fact a physician has to be both realist and nominalists. He must study the individual as well as the disease. . . . Medicine should not be likened to any science. Physicians have to face both concrete reality and scientific abstractions. Their mind must simultaneously grasp the phenomena and their symbols, search into organs and consciousness, and enter,

11

with each individual, a different world. They are asked to realize the impossible feat of building up *a science of the particular*. (Abridged, pp. 246–249; emphasis added)

The next bold step Szasz took was his 1961 book bearing the same title as the 1960 paper stating his purpose as follows: "The question 'What *is* mental illness?' is shown to be inextricably linked to the question 'What do psychiatrists do?'"; this was sound operationalism as once defined for physics by Bridgman (1927) and Einstein:

> If you want to find out anything from the theoretical physicists about the methods they use, I advise you to stick closely to one principle: Don't listen to their words, fix you attention on their deeds. (p. 30) (Szasz, 1961, p. 2)

Furthermore, Szasz declared,

> since it is difficult to scrap one conceptual model without having another with which to replace it, . . . my second task is to offer a "constructive" synthesis of knowledge . . . Although my thesis is that mental illness is a myth, this book is not an attempt to "debunk psychiatry" . . . I believe that psychiatry could be a science. I also believe that psychotherapy is an effective method of helping people— not to recover from an "illness," it is true, but rather to learn about themselves, others, and life (pp. x–xi).

These cautionary words were not heeded by those who attacked Szasz; he envisioned a science based on language, interpersonal communication by means of speech acts and informed by ethics.

Hysteria as Freud's and Szasz's Model of Disorder and Lothane's Dramatology

Szasz's incisive critique of psychiatry and psychoanalysis focused on the label hysteria: what it was and is and what was done with it. Again, let us first take a look at the label itself. Whereas Hippocrates held that "the womb, *hystera*, is the origin of all disease" there is no noun hysteria in Hippocrates only the adjective *histerike pnix*, or hysterical suffocation of the womb. Plato allegorized, dramatized, and personified the womb as "an animal desirous of procreating children and when remaining unfruitful gets discontented and angry and wandering in every direction through the body, closes up the passages of the breath, and by obstructing respiration, drives the women to extremity, causing all varieties of disease" (Lothane, 1995). Although antithetical to science,

12

myths do reveal truths about life as well: just replace womb with woman and you realize that the woman's tasks are copulation, procreation, and child rearing, the same as suggested by myths of Paradise and the Fall. While the adjective hysterical was used in English in the seventeenth and eighteenth centuries, the noun became naturalized following its scientific use in French as *hystérie*. Hysterectomy still means removing the womb even though there is no gynecological disease called hysteria. Second, Freud and Breuer (1895) used both the adjective hysterical, for example, hysterical phenomena, and the noun hysteria, for example, the psychotherapy of hysteria.

For Szasz the label hysteria became the paradigm of mental illness, the pivot debate, and the straw man: he got some issues right and misunderstood others. The main thing he got right was that the patient's so-called symptoms, under the sway of the medical model, were actually *communications* to self and others and *conducts*, not conditions, an idea that had already been articulated in 1951, ten years before Szasz, by Ruesch and Bateson, and duly cited by Szasz in 1961. Still bound to the medical model, Freud codified that so-called hysterics, for example, people who complained of having paralyses or being paralyzed, were showing functional, that is, unreal paralyses but *no* organic, or real, paralyses. The truth was that they showed neither organic nor nonorganic paralyses, they showed no paralyses at all, they were people *impersonating* paralytics who *dramatized* their painful conflicts and crises in pantomimic body language, in words, and emotions (Lothane, 2009, 2010a). The task of the psychosocially oriented doctor was to *translate* the *manifest* verbal and nonverbal communications, whose traumatic meanings remained unknown to the patients because they used repression as a defense to avoid or anesthetize the pain, back to their *latent* or hidden meanings and to memories of traumas, expressible in everyday language, dynamics Breuer and Freud described in 1895 in their epochal *Studies on Hysteria* and Freud in his 1900 *The Interpretation of Dreams*. It was a kind of a confrontation with the truth of their emotional experiences versus strategies of evasion of that truth by means of dramatization in act and in fantasy. The further corollary of that insight was that the so-called symptoms of hysteria were dramatic enactments and that these were structured like dreams, with a manifest and latent content.

It was Breuer, as I found (Lothane, 2009), who wrote that his famous patient Anna O's *dramatized* (lost in the Strachey-Tyson translation) her thoughts and emotions in enactments. It was Szasz who found that

13

Breuer had called her enactments "masquerades" to which Szasz added charades (Szasz, 1961, p. 298). Such enactments are not phony, only their attribution to organic illness is phony: in themselves these acts as communications are amenable to being analyzed and understood not only via empathy, a function of sympathy or the emotional contact with the other, but also with the help of a technique Freud learned from interpreting dreams, that is, free association. I believe Freud and Szasz would have approved of my concept of *dramatology* (Lothane, 2009, 2010), an approach encompassing dramatization in fantasy, action, and interaction, that is, verbal and gestural communication, a new heuristic addition to the psychoanalytic method (Lothane, 2007a, 2007b, 2009, 2010a, 2010b, 2011a). As Szasz noted in his 2008 book: "the problem was drama, not disease" (p. 26). The conclusion we share is this: the disease called hysteria is just a traditional label affixed to certain aspects of the dramas of life, a *flatus vocis*, with implications for other forms of disordered conduct.

Certain self-contradictions in Freud are traceable to Freud himself who tended to conflate his revolutionary psychoanalytic *method*, a small portion of his output, with his *theories* of disorder, the lion's share of his collected works. This conflation has persisted ever since in the psychoanalytic literature. It cannot be emphasized enough: Freud's method of treatment was *always* dyadic, that is, interpersonal and interactional, but in his theories of disorder he still adhered to monadic definitions, to mixing psychology with physiology, or exegetics with energetic, as in the libido theory of sexuality, a topic Szasz had written very little about. Szasz repeated this conflation when he claimed incorrectly that "Breuer and Freud (1895, pp. xxii, xxiv, xxix) [entertained] partly 'organic' hypotheses for the cause 'cause' of this 'disease'" (1961, p. 80): the pages cited are not the opinions of the Breuer and Freud but editorial comments of translators Strachey and Tyson; this was not Freud toying with any "Cartesian dualism" (p. 78). Nor was Freud doing the above with his theory on conversion hysteria: there was no "jumping from the psychic into the organic" in the case of "a young lady . . . [with] pains in her legs and who had difficulties walking" (p. 79); rather, as in an earlier statement by Freud Szasz quoted, so-called conversion was "a 'symbolic' relation . . . [like] vomiting upon a feeling of moral disgust" (p. 79), a prima facie case of expressing *emotions*. There was no more "conversion" in the so-called hysteric than in any person lifting an arm or choosing not to lift it. No hysteria, no conversion, no need to belabor the point: it is but a *façon de parler*. A thornier issue for Szasz was bodily manifestations of the psychosomatic kind, for example, experiencing fear and expressing it with a bout of a transient vomiting or diarrhea, not enough to diagnose any organic disorder, but a lot of feelings and emotions (Lothane, 2014). I submit that it was Szasz's occasional Cartesian dualism that made him shy away from psychosomatics and engage in polemics with the other great Hungarian, the head of psychoanalysis in Chicago, Franz Alexander.

Szasz repeatedly juxtaposed "typical organic disease, . . . [which] is not autobiographical, [whose] symptoms are anatomically and physiologically determined" (1961, p. 136), that is, real illness, and the various fake forms of "illness," continuing to excoriate Freud for his "characteristically deceptive rhetoric, treating persons as objects, the vehicles and victims of mental diseases, and psychiatric-psychoanalytic abstractions as personalized agents with the power to *counterfeit* organic nervous disorders" (p. 40). First, even though Freud occasionally mixed organic and functional language, he also unequivocally transitioned from medicine and biology to psychology and sociology. Rather than making the case for interpersonal psychoanalysis by the just mentioned juxtaposition, Szasz should have remained focused on analyzing *from within* the methods and politics of psychiatry itself, from its beginnings.

Some Lessons of the History of Psychiatry

Psychiatry began at the start of the nineteenth century with Pinel not toward the end of the nineteenth century as Szasz has it: it was only psychoanalysis that was born at the end of the nineteenth century. Furthermore, it was not Pinel's apocryphal gesture of liberating the insane from their chains that did it but learning from the couple Pussin, who ran the Bicêtre Asylum in Paris and who had started that liberation, but Pinel's medicalization of the existing so-called maisons de santé, or asylums, and making psychiatry both a new medical discipline and a social institution.

The first psychiatric century began with Philippe Pinel's (1801) *A Treatise on Insanity* ending in 1899 with the publication of two epochal works: Emil Kraepelin's 6th edition of his *Textbook of Psychiatry* and Sigmund Freud's *Interpretation of Dreams* (postdated by the publisher to 1900 to celebrate the 20th century). Philippe Pinel (1745–1826), originally a professor of medicine, founded psychiatry as a profession that promised power, profit and prestige to its practitioners. Pinel divided the profession into academic psychiatry at university centers and institutional psychiatry in rural and urban areas. Pinel's classification of disorders was limited and he regarded disordered conduct as largely due to social and psychological causes and thus amenable to "moral treatment," that is, persuasion and psychotherapy. (Lothane, 2011b)

Psychiatry evolved as follows:

In the course of that history two major conceptions of the nature and treatment of psychosocial disorders called neuroses and psychoses emerged, the *somatic* or biological and the *dynamic*, or psychological and social, also called psychodynamic. In the first half of the 19th century the leading representatives of the dynamic conception were Philippe Pinel and Jean-Etienne Esquirol in France and Johann Christian Reil and Johann Christian August Heinroth in Germany, the latter collectively called the *Psychiker*, distinct from the *Somatiker*, the psychological psychiatrists and the biological psychiatrists, respectively. In the second half of the 19th century, the German psychiatrist Wilhelm Griesinger still combined both approaches, but his 1845 dictum that "mental diseases are brain diseases" paved the way for the ultimate victory of the *Somatiker* over the *Psychiker* and the rise of "an overall system of organic and mechanistic psychiatry" (Ellenberger, 1970, p. 284), coercive and often cruel, using somatic treatments such as drugs, bed rest and isolation, hydrotherapy and electrotherapy, with little or no recourse to psychotherapy. The somatic, as an organ and body oriented approach, had its roots in the millennia-long tradition of medicine which examined the sick body and treated it with drugs and surgery. Even as Emil Kraepelin (1856–1926) was seen by Ellenberger as caring and utilizing multiple approaches to psychopathology, his system of psychiatry was predominantly descriptive and static. The tradition of the *Psychiker* made a comeback in the late 1880's with two Swiss psychiatrists, the founders of the Zurich school of psychiatry. The first was Auguste-Henri Forel (1848–1931), the teacher of the Swiss-born Adolf Meyer (1866–1950), and an early champion of psychodynamic ideas psychoanalysis in the United States. The second was Eugen Bleuler (1857–1939), successor of Forel as director of the famed Burghölzli asylum, the first in 1896 to endorse Sigmund Freud's (1856–1939) epochal *Studies on Hysteria* in 1896, who conducted experimental studies of thought association and promoted psychoanalytically-based psychotherapy in the treatment of psychotic patients. By 1900 the Zurich school gained an important member: Carl Gustav Jung (1875–1961). Bleuler and Jung were the first, if not the only ones, to give early scientific recognition to psychoanalysis in German-speaking countries. (Lothane, 2011c)

Freud made no mention of dynamic psychiatry in the first half of the nineteenth century. Even though both famous Swiss psychiatrists'

Eugen Bleuler and Adolf Meyer approach to schizophrenia could be viewed from the perspective of Meyer's inclusive term psychobiology, it was ultimately Kraepelin who turned out to be the victor and inspiration for the American DSM's III, IV, and V and the European ICD's nomenclatures. Kraepelin achieved the feat of giving a final shape to descriptive psychiatry when he converted thousands of individual observations and narratives, recorded on those legendary index cards (*Zählkarten*) by means of abstraction, generalization, and schematization, into his new taxonomy of psychiatric diseases, starting with the first edition of his *Textbook* in 1883. At the same time, as a student of Wilhelm Wundt, he was more psychologically minded than his contemporaries and thus initially aware, in the fifth edition, that "it is impossible make a radical separation between healthy and morbid states, . . . between all the possible transitional forms in life and the particular scientifically-derived 'disease-forms' . . . Therefore, for now and perhaps forever, we must refrain from a simple classification of mental disorders in the manner of Linné and scientifically-defined types" (Kraepelin, 1896, p. 312; my translations throughout). In the sixth edition of his *Textbook* Kraepelin's method and system were fully codified and applied to the diagnosing and treatment of psychiatric inpatients. But here is the crux of the problem: the conditions and goals of inpatient treatment (intra muros, within the walls of the asylum) are vastly different from the conditions and goals of private practice (extra muros outside the walls, in the doctor's office). One of Freud's insufficiently recognized contributions to psychiatry was to lay down the foundation and method of an autonomous psychotherapy, as Szasz would later call it. It should be remembered that it was Freud's psychoanalytic movement that played a role in the expansion and growth of outpatient practice, starting in Vienna and pursued in other places by forgotten pioneers such as Ludwig Binswanger, Poul Bjerre, Alphonse Maeder, and Jung himself. Kraepelin's method was an inspiration for Karl Jaspers, author for the most influential psychiatric textbook in Germany and beyond (Jaspers, 1973). Szasz did not confront Jaspers' rigid and static organicism and his repudiation of Freud's dynamic approach to hallucinations and delusions. The latter brings me to Freud and Schreber (Lothane, 1992). Before we discuss Freud and Schreber here is a bit of history about the psychiatric approach to hallucinations:

Before Kraepelin *Psychiker* Leubuscher (1852) argued from a perspective of the person that since the senses as such do not deceive, we should actually speak of *deceptions through the senses* (p. 2) These develop through 1) the *involuntary* process of the *fantasy* play of *ideas*; 2) an emotion or a passion; 3) the will, or an intention directed or fixated on an image (p. 27). The latter form of hallucinations could be described as *psychic* . . . produced by psychic causes . . . often showing the *condensation* of an idea floating over time" (p. 32; emphasis his). Retreating from the aforementioned position on auditory hallucinations, Kraepelin classified hallucinations, a basic "phenomenon of insanity," under the rubric of "*disorders of the organs of perception*." Jaspers (1973) went him one better in his idiosyncratic *Phänomenologie* defining hallucinations as "elementary phenomena," "Ur-phenomena," as "the basic units of consciousness-of-existence considered in isolation, e.g., hallucinations, feeling states, drive-impulses" (p. 49). Jaspers reified an elementary phenomenon, a kind of a psychological atom, ripped it from the fullness of apprehending the world perceptually, imaginatively, and emotionally, promoting a dubious explanatory science while denying Freud's depth psychology. He created a soulless and sterile system that paved the way for jurist Binding and psychiatrist Hoche (1920) to champion euthanasia of mental patients. It reached its horrific climax during the Nazi regime when Sonnenstein, no longer an asylum, became one of the euthanasia sites of chronic patients and Soviet POW's, under its medical director Dr. Nitzsche, tried, convicted and executed for crimes against humanity (Böhm, 2000). Sonnenstein now houses a museum of and memorial to the martyrs. Their murders were a dress rehearsal for Auschwitz. (Friedlander, 1995) (Lothane, 2011b)

The error of defining hallucinations as disorders of perception (Lothane, 1982) has been perpetuated in nomenclatures and psychiatric textbooks. For Kraepelin and his followers hallucinations and delusions were primary manifestations of psychosis, for Bleuler these were secondary manifestations, thus not a criterion for prima facie diagnosing either schizophrenia or manic-depressive psychosis.

Szasz and My Work on Schreber

Szasz's libertarian ideas about coercive hospitalization of mental patients influenced my work on Schreber. In his 1911 analysis of Schreber's book, since Freud never met Schreber, Freud utilized a number of approaches. On the one hand, he applied the transformative dynamics of the dream: the dream work (*Traumarbeit*) is paralleled by delusion-work (*Wahnarbeit*) and hallucination-work. On the other hand, he focused on Schreber's alleged homosexual desires. However, Freud overlooked his original insight, that both the manifest neurosis and the manifest dream are caused by recent trauma of adult life or by remote trauma of childhood; that in both the manifest content is a transformation, or a translation, of the language of everyday life into the language of fantasy and fulfillment of wishes, as compensation for the traumatic/dramatic conflict and emotional pain. In addition, both are the dream and neurosis are a historical record of a life, both decodable by overcoming resistance, free association, and interpretation.

Instead of following the dream and drama method, Freud declared he "had developed [his] theory of paranoia before [he] became acquainted with the contents of Schreber's book" (p. 79), that is, applied to Schreber a preformed *formula*. He cited a 1908 paper by Abraham, Jung's 1907 book *The Psychology of Dementia praecox*, the second psychiatrist to discuss the Schreber case in the literature, and admitted that "Abraham's short paper contains almost all the essential views put forward in the present study of the case of Schreber" (Footnote 1, p. 70). The result was a deplorable mish-mash of mistaken diagnoses and an erroneous dynamics: Schreber was neither paranoid, paraphrenic, nor schizophrenic, he suffered from a mood disorder. As to Freud's interpretation that Schreber became ill due to his homosexual desire to have his psychiatrist Flechsig penetrate him anally Jung had this to say: "Only now that I have the galleys can I enjoy your Schreber. It is not only uproariously funny but brilliantly written as well. If I were an altruist I would now be saying how glad I am that you have taken Schreber under your wing and shown psychiatry what treasures are heaped up there. But, as it is, I must content myself with the invidious role I got in there first . . ." (*Freud/Jung Letters*, p. 407). But Jung was there first: why didn't he go on to write his own thesis on Schreber?

I interpreted Schreber's fantasy of turning into a woman not as a homosexual wish but an identification with a child-bearing woman as compensation for his thwarted desires to have children due to his wife's repeated miscarriages and stillborn babies, the last, a boy, in 1892, prior to the onset of his agitated and suicidal depression in 1893, the traumatic reaction which was the main event in his book. For Freud paranoia was still an *intrapersonal* fact. Seen interpersonally, it takes one person to develop pneumonia, it takes two to develop paranoia. Schreber's "paranoia" toward Flechsig was the accusation of malpractice as abandonment. Schreber did not express any paranoid ideas toward his real persecutor, Weber, and argued against him as follows: "The only difference of opinion is whether the subjective sensation of hearing voices is caused only by pathological functioning of my

19

nerves . . . or whether some being outside my body speaks to me in the form of voices. . . . *In essence it is one assertion versus another*" (Schreber, 1903, pp. 418–419; emphasis Schreber's), denying Weber the authority to declare him insane. It has been observed many times: one man's mythology is another man's pathology.

Whereas Freud caved in both to Kraepelin's ideas and to the diagnosis of paranoia made by Schreber's jailer, Sonnenstein director Guido Weber, Schreber (1903), who in his capacity as judge was acquainted with clinical and forensic psychiatry, engaged in a debate with Kraepelin:

> Schreber had some inkling of unconscious truth: "I believe there is a grain of truth in most folklore, some presentiment of supernatural matters which in the course of time have dawned on a large number of people, naturally much augmented by deliberate elaboration of man's fantasy, so that the grain of truth can now hardly be shelled out" (p. 339), thus, perhaps (a word Schreber used repeatedly), "after all there was some truth in my so-called delusions and hallucinations" (p. 123, footnote #63). Such beliefs expressed in concealed form Schreber's emotional reality. (Lothane, 2011b)

Schreber (1903) rebutted Kraepelin as follows:

> I noticed with great interest that according to Kraepelin's *Textbook of Psychiatry* (5th Edition, Leipzig 1896 p. 95ff.) the phenomenon of being in some supernatural communication with voices had frequently been observed before in humans whose nerves were in a state of morbid excitation. I do not dispute that in many of these cases one may only be dealing with mere hallucinations, as they are treated throughout the mentioned textbook. In my opinion science would go very wrong to designate as 'hallucinations' *all* such phenomena that lack objective reality (pp. 89-90); A person with sound nerves is, so to speak, *mentally* blind compared with him who receives supernatural impression by virtue of his diseased nerves; he is therefore as little likely to persuade the visionary of the unreality of his visions as person who can see will be persuaded by a really blind person that there are no colours, that blue is not blue, red not red, etc. (p. 224; Schreber's italics); I think it is quite possible that some such cases were instances of genuine seers of spirits . . . Even so-called spiritualist mediums may be considered genuine seers of spirits of the inferior kind in this sense, although in many cases self-deception and fraud may also play a part. Therefore one ought to beware of unscientific generalizations and rash condemnation in such matters. If psychiatry is not to deny everything supernatural and thus tumble with both feet into the camp of naked materialism, it will have to recognize the possibility that occasionally the phenomena under discussion may be connected with real happenings, which simply cannot be brushed aside with the catchword 'hallucinations.' (p. 90)

Similar claims were made by other former inpatients who claimed that important mystical insights were vouchsafed to them during psychotic episodes, for example, psychiatrist Boisen (1936, 1960) and layman Custance (1952, 1954). The question remains, how does one go about certifying a genuine mystic? One might find some answers by consulting the Prophet Ezekiel, St. John of the Cross, St. Teresa of Avila, and St. Joan of Arc, the last mentioned by Schreber; and also Hildegard von Bingen, Mechthild von Magdeburg, Jakob Böhme, all cited by Buber (1923); or the Jewish kabbalistic mystics cited by Scholem (1941) (Lothane, 2011b). And one cannot deny legitimacy to some ideas in Schreber's private religion.

Schreber's purpose of writing his book was to prove his sanity and get back his freedom and civil rights after eight years of psychiatric incarceration against his will, as he expressed in the title of his essay on forensic psychiatry: "In what circumstances can a person considered insane be detained in asylum against his declared will?" (1903, pp. 363–376), which was also the subtitle of his book, left untranslated by Macalpine and Hunter (Schreber, 1955); moreover, they obliterated Schreber as the *author* who had worthy reflections about being labeled as paranoid by changing Schreber's title to memoirs about an illness. Freud, too, was now aware of how the conditions of hospitalization affected the content and intent of Schreber's so-called hallucinations and delusions.

Since my first publication on Schreber in 1989 I have steadily defended Schreber's father and son against various historical mistakes and biased misreadings. In 2011 I received the Thomas S. Szasz award "For outstanding contributions to the cause of civil liberties." I claim two contributions: defending Schreber and interceding for eighteen-year-old Richard who was my patient many years ago in an open psychiatric hospital. His father wanted him committed to a state hospital and I prevented it and the patient was placed in a residence. For many years now he calls on the phone to thank me for having saved his life. He usually tells me he loves me and promises to come and visit, but never does and I doubt if he ever will but I duly reciprocate with my good wishes to him.

What is in a name? A rose by any other name would smell as sweet. Mental illness is a name, the reality it refers to is not just problems in living but more acutely, problems caused by destructive antisocial or criminal conduct by persons both sane and insane. As society's institutions, law and psychiatry cannot avoid coercion and join forces in maintaining law and order and remanding trouble-makers either

21

to prisons or hospitals in lieu of prisons. John Hinckley Jr., would be assassin of Reagan, benefited from being sent to St. Elizabeth hospital rather than a prison.

Szasz did not destroy psychiatry in New York State or anywhere else, he was only a voice of conscience and criticism, something every discipline needs. The mammoth state hospitals like Pilgrim State Hospital on Long Island, associated with memories of *The Snake Pit* and *Titicut Follies*, were emptied following the rise of community psychiatry and because New York State could no longer afford them. Like Freud before him, Szasz made a lasting contribution to humanizing psychiatry. Both Freud and Szasz were unusually gifted writers who knew how to put things across with word magic, with words that held no punches and drove the point home with a felicitous turn of speech and at times with hyperbole for extra emphasis. They spoke of science with respect but identified strongly with literary geniuses that preceded them. Freud's claim that all feelings were sexual and gadfly Szasz calling mental illness a myth and a lie were meant to épater les bourgeois, to shock ingrained habits of dealing with patients, to stir professionals to self-reflection and change. Their words were not meant to incite to acts of destruction, hatred or revenge but rather were spoken or written with a tongue in cheek attitude bred of a kind of irony practiced earlier by another famous atheistic Jew, Heinrich Heine, who died the year Freud was born: "God will forgive me," quoth Heine in French on his death bed, "he does this for a living." Or we might even reach into earlier history and remember the other social gadfly, Socrates, who sought to define the form of the good while suggesting that an unexamined life is not worth living but ended drinking the deadly draft of hemlock as the price for defending his ideas.

References

Breuer, J., & Freud, S. (1895). *Studies on hysteria*. Standard Edition, 2. London: Hogarth Press.

Bridgman, P. W. (1927). *The logic of modern physics*. New York: Macmillan.

Carrel, A. (1935). *Man the unknown*. New York and London: Harper & Brothers.

Ellenberger, H. (1970). *The discovery of the unconscious: The history and evolution of dynamic psychiatry*. New York: Basic Books, Inc.

Freud, S. (1911). *Psycho-analytic notes on an autobiographical account of a case of paranoia (dementia paranoides)*. SE, 12: 9–82.

Freud, S. (1933 [1932]). *Why war?* Standard Edition, 22: 199–215.

Freud, S. (1974). *The jung letters*. Edited by William McGuire. Princeton, NJ: Princeton Univesity Press.

Freud, S. (1900). *The interpretation of dreams*. Standard Edition, 4, 5.

Glaser, F. B. (1965). The dichotomy game a further consideration of the writings of Dr. Thomas Szasz. *American Journal of Psychiatry, 121*(11), 1069–1074.

Goffman, E. (1961). *Asylums: Essays on the social situation of mental patients and other inmates*. New York: Anchor Books.

Jaspers, K. (1973). *Allgemeine Psychopathologie* (general psychopathology). Neunte, unververänderte Auflage. Berlin: Springer Verlag.

Kraepelin, E. (1896). *Psychiatrie ein lehrbuch für studirende und aerzte* (a textbook for students and doctors). Leipzig: Barth.

Lothane, Z. (1982). The psychopathology of hallucinations—A methodological analysis. *British Journal of Medical Psychology, 55*, 339–348.

Lothane, Z. (1992). *In defense of Schreber: Soul murder and psychiatry*. Hillsdale, NJ and London: The Psychoanalytic Press.

Lothane, Z. (1995). Hysteria beyond Freud. Review of *Hysteria beyond Freud* by Sander L. Gilman, H. King, Roy Porter, G. S. Rousseau & E. Showalter Berkeley: California University Press, 1993. *Psychoanalytic Books, 6*(1), 74–87.

Lothane, Z. (2007a). The power of the spoken word in life, psychiatry and psychoanalysis—A contribution to interpersonal psychoanalysis. *American Journal of Psychoanalysis, 67*, 260–274.

Lothane, Z. (2007b). Imagination as a reciprocal process and its role in the psychoanalytic situation. *International Forum of Psychoanalysis, 16*, 152–163.

Lothane, Z. (2009). Dramatology in life, disorder, and psychoanalytic therapy: A further contribution to interpersonal psychoanalysis. *International Forum of Psychoanalysis, 18*, 135–148.

Lothane, Z. (2010a). Dramatology: A new paradigm for psychiatry and psychotherapy. *Psychiatric Times*, June 2010, 22–23.

Lothane, Z. (2010b). The analyst and analyst team practicing reciprocal free association—Defenders and deniers. *International Forum of Psychoanalysis, 19*, 1–10.

Lothane, H. Z. (2011a). Dramatology vs. narratology: A new synthesis for psychiatry, psychoanalysis, and interpersonal drama therapy (IDT). *Archives of Psychiatry and Psychotherapy, 4*, 29–43.

Lothane, Z. (2011b). The teachings of honorary professor of psychiatry Daniel Paul Schreber J.D. to psychiatrists and psychoanalysts, or dramatology's challenge to psychiatry and psychoanalysis. *The Psychoanalytic Review, 98*(6), 775–815.

Lothane, Z. (2011c). The partnership of psychoanalysis and psychiatry in the treatment of psychosis and borderline states: Its evolution in North America. *Journal of the American Academy of Psychoanalysis and Dynamic Psychiatry, 39*(3), 499–524.

Lothane, H. Z. (2012). Dr Thomas Szasz psychiatrist and psychoanalyst who challenged the medical world with deeply unconventional views on the nature of mental illness. London: *The Times*, Thursday October 11 2012 No 70701. http://www.thetimes.co.uk/tto/opinion/obituaries/article3564350.ece

Lothane, H. Z. (2014). Emotional reality: A further contribution to dramatology. *International Forum of Psychoanalysis*. doi:10.1080/0803706X.2014.953996

Pleune, G. F. (1965). All dis-ease is not disease: A consideration of psychoanalysis, psychotherapy, and psycho-social engineering. *International Journal of Psycho-Analysis, 46*, 358–366.

Ruesch, J., & Bateson, G. (1951). *Communication: The social matrix of psychiatry.* New York: Norton.

Schaler, J. A. (Ed.). (2004). *Szasz under fire: The psychiatric abolitionist faces his critics.* Chicago and La Salle, IL: Open Court.

Schreber, D. P. (1903). *Denkwürdigkeiten eines Nervenkranken nebst Nachträge und einem Anhang über die Frage:«Unter welchen Voraussetzungen darf eine für geisteskrank erachtete Person gegen ihren erklärten Willen in eine Heilanstalt festgehalten werden?»* (reflections of a nervous patient with addenda and a supplement concerning the question: "Under what premises may a person considered insane be held in an asylum against his declared will?" Leipzig: Mutze.

Schreber, D. P. (1955). *Memoirs of my nervous illness* (I. Macalpine & R. A. Hunter, Trans & Ed.). London: Dawson.

Szasz, T. S. (1960). The myth of mental illness. *The American Psychologist, 15*(2), 113–118.

Szasz, T. S. (1961). *The myth of mental illness: Foundations of a theory of personal conduct.* New York: A Hoeber-Harper Book.

Szasz, T. S. (1965). *The ethics of psychoanalysis: The theory and method of autonomous psychotherapy.* New York: Basic Books.

Szasz, T. S. (2008). *Psychiatry: The science of lies.* Syracuse: Syracuse University Press.

2

In Dialogue with Thomas Szasz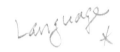

Susan Petrilli and Augusto Ponzio

p. 208

Remembering the First Time We Met . . .

We met Thomas S. Szasz personally for the first time in November 2003 at the International Congress *Medicina e humanitas* (Medecine and humanitas), hosted by the Università del Secondo Rinascimento, organized at the Villa Borromeo (Senago, Milan) by Armando Verdiglione and Cristina Frua De Angelis. For the occasion, Szasz delivered a paper entitled "Why I wrote *The Myth of Mental Illness*."

We were struck by the humility that characterized such a preeminent figure and by his readiness to listen. And yet he was among the most renowned authors of the twentieth century—thanks especially to *The Myth of Mental Illness*, his book of 1961 (revised editions 1974, 2010), which in 2003 was launched in a new Italian edition with Spirali Edizioni (Milan). Many other writings by Szasz had already appeared over the preceding decade in Italian translation with the same publisher.

Szasz's special interests led to his focus on problematics connected with signs, language and communication. He was convinced that a good theory of the subject required a good linguistic theory, a good theory of sign and of language.

Consequently, he was keen to accept our invitation to hold a seminar on the relationship between subjectivity, language, and the body at the University of Bari Aldo Moro, for our courses in semiotics and philosophy of language and for our Ph.D. program in "Language Theory and the Sign Sciences." It was agreed that we would organize the event within a few months thereafter.

In fact the meeting took place on 18 May, 2004, under the title *Protolinguaggio, il linguaggio del corpo* (Protolanguage, body language).

It turned out to be a real conference with the participation not only of our PhD students, but also of colleagues from different disciplines and surrounding universities. The climate was intense with expectation and enthusiasm. The general discussion provoked by the lesson delivered by Szasz was extraordinarily lively and saw the participation of all those present. The results of this meeting, a text by Szasz presented with comments from the debate, were published in Italian in *PLAT, Quaderni del dipartimento di Pratiche linguistiche e Analisi di Testi* (Workbooks of the Department of Linguistic Practices and Text Analysis) (3, 2004, pp. 9–24). The year before we had already published another brief text by Szasz in Italian translation in our journal *Corposcritto* (4, 2003, pp. 137–143), "Se vogliamo parlare senza infingimenti del suicidio" ("Straight Talk about Suicide"). We were rehearsing unaware for an act that was to take place a few years later, the Italian translation of a book by Szasz that did not yet exist, but that was surely on its way, *"My Madness saved Me": The Madness and Marriage of Virginia Woolf*, with Transaction Publishers, 2006.

The present text coauthored by Susan Petrilli and Augusto Ponzio is divided into three parts: this initial part, " Remembering the First Time We Met . . .", serves as an introduction to the two that follow; "From Translating Him to Participating with His Word," by Susan Petrilli; and "Reading Virginia's Word with Him," by Augusto Ponzio. They have been conceived together as a unitary text.

In particular: in the part immediately following on from the present, Susan Petrilli, who was committed to translating Thomas Szasz's book on Virginia Woolf (from English into Italian), discusses certain aspects of the question of translation with special reference to Szasz. In the first place translation involves the practice of listening to the other and listening is the necessary condition for successful communication in general. This emerges ever more clearly when we engage in transferring a text from one historical-natural language to another. In the process, meanings are amplified and enhanced: the work of translation is also the work of interpretation, typical of the psychoanalytical session which too demands listening as its unconditional basis.

In "dialogue" with Szasz we explore such concepts as "language," "dialogism," "utterance," "encounter," listening," "responsibility" and "otherness." The relationship with the other as thematized in sign, language and communication theory is no less than central in the development of the human psyche as much as it is in language and communication, in fact is constitutive of the former. It is with respect to this theme in particular that encounter is achieved between Szasz and his overall conception and our own as elaborated in our preceding works, both individual—and they are not few—as well as those written in collaboration.

With the conceptual instruments of the sign and language sciences we examine such issues as the claim made by Szasz that mental illness is a metaphor, the problem of subjectivity, of identity, the distinction between conscious and unconscious life, the problem of understanding, of dialogue, and of what Szasz likes to call "self-conversation." Particularly interesting is the relationship that can be established between what is commonly discredited as the "pathological condition" of "hearing voices" and the happy condition of "dialogized plurilingualism," as theorized by Mikhail Bakhtin and taken into consideration on several occasions by Szasz himself. The question of identity is examined in this framework, occasioned by Szasz's monograph on Virginia Woolf and the fuzzy distinction between "madness" and "genius."

In the part signed specifically by Augusto Ponzio a special focus is placed on a concept that is central both in a book of 1996 by Szasz entitled *The Meaning of Mind: Language, Morality, and Neuroscience* as well as in his book on Virginia Woolf. The concept is that of "moral agent." In Ponzio's view, a substantialist perspective persists in this notion, as though there were a subject, in the sense of *subjectus, substans*, upon which there stand a series of qualities, behaviors, decisional acts managed by that subject. But there is no such thing as a subject a priori with respect to the act, the linguistic act, with respect to the word, whether interior or exterior. Just as there is no such thing as an author taken separately from his existence in the text. Therefore, Virginia Woolf comes to life at each occurrence in her writings. Not only in her literary writings, but also in her "private" writings, in her diaries, in her letters. Subjectivity cannot be considered as something that is pregiven, preconstituted, pre-established once and for all.

Szasz throughout all his works beginning from *The Myth of Mental Illness* criticized the belief that there are people who are healthy minded and people who are mentally ill, on which basis behavior is then described as normal or pathological. Yet, despite this we can make the claim that in Szasz, in his concept of "moral agent," there still persists the attribution to the individual of a preconstituted identity, given which there ensue certain behaviors, decisions, and preferences.

This does not take away from the inevitable fascination and strong involvement elicited no doubt by all of Szasz's work, but perhaps above

27

all by this book on Virginia Woolf; and this may be the case here because Thomas Szasz is dealing with literary writing and what's more with the writing of a writer considered a "mad-genius".

From Translating to Participating with His Word—Susan Petrilli

Each large and creative verbal whole is a very complex and multifaceted system of relations. With a creative attitude toward language, there are no voiceless words that belong to no one. Each word contains voices that are sometimes infinitely distant, unnamed, almost impersonal (voices of lexical shadings, of styles, and so forth), almost undetectable, and voices resounding nearby and simultaneously (Mikhail M. Bakhtin, 1986, p. 124).

Dialogue and dialectics. Take a dialogue and remove the voices (the partitioning of voices), remove the intonations (emotional and individualizing ones), carve out abstract concepts and judgments from living words and responses, cram everything into one abstract consciousness—and that's how you get dialectics (Bakhtin, 1986, p. 147).

Listening as the Condition for Speaking and Encounter

Translating Thomas Szasz's book on Virginia Woolf into Italian for publication with Spirali (*La mia follia mi ha salvato. La follia e il matrimonio di Virginia Woolf*) was an extraordinary experience and truly engaging. It was the first time I was reading this author so closely.

The title "*My Madness Saved Me*": *The Madness and Marriage of Virginia Woolf* was intriguing in itself and stimulated my curiosity beyond my consolidated interest in Szasz and his writings. My immediate response was the desire to translate this book into Italian.

Translation from one language to another: this is a way of listening to the word of the other and of reading while writing and writing while reading. To translate is to connect with the other, to travel with the other and engage in the unending search for sense—of words, narrations, lived experiences, relationships. In this journey nothing can be taken for granted, nothing is simple, and yet it seduces and is vital. Translation evidences how the text continuously generates new signs and senses that dialogue with each other, complementary and accomplices in the construction of new worlds. This is to say that all efforts made by the writer/interpreter/translator to unravel the sense of the text, reaching for clarity and explanation inevitably generate new spheres of signification, new interpretive itineraries with the possibility of new and enhanced understanding of the text in translation.

Thematization of language is a constant in writings by Szasz, wherein nothing is taken for granted. His book on Virginia Woolf, a book of reflections and analyses on problems of life, communication and relationships, is strongly dialogical. Here our allusion is to dialogue in the theatrical sense of the term, that is, representation of the relationship with the other. Dialogism in Szasz is not at all of the formal order; that is, dialogue understood in the formal sense of the exchange of rejoinders. Such exchange does not necessarily imply real interaction, listening, and participation on the part of all interlocutors involved. Rather, in Szasz's interpretation dialogue is understood in the sense of *encounter*, and this occurs and is made possible on the basis of *listening*. This is one of the reasons why this particular book by Szasz can be described as a complex book, precisely because it is structured according to different levels of experience and discourse, characterized by the will to raise questions about life and relationships without ever claiming to know all the answers.

Initially, the statement that mental illness does not exist appeared rather disconcerting to me. However, I soon realized that Szasz was saying something else that was very interesting, namely that mental illness is predicated about the body. Consequently, when we speak about "mental illness," we are applying a concept of the physical order to the "mind"—another concept that needed to be questioned, as we shall see below. Therefore, the expression "mental illness" is a metaphor, as he claimed in his very first book of 1961, *The Myth of Mental Illness*, and as he repeats in chapter 6, "Modernity's Master Metaphors: Mental Illness and Mental Treatment," of his 1996 book, *The Meaning of Mind: Language, Morality, and Neuroscience* and as well as in numerous other venues, including books, articles, speeches, and media appearances. This statement is the main axiom around which Szasz developed his whole vision of psychiatry and psychiatrists. From the Preface to the second 1974 edition of his *Myth of Mental Illness* (the last was in 2010):

> I maintain that mental illness is a metaphorical disease: that bodily illness stands in the same relation to mental illness as a defective television to a bad television program. Of course, the word "sick" is often used metaphorically. We call jokes "sick," economies "sick," sometimes even the whole world "sick"; but only when we call minds "sick" do we systematically mistake and strategically misinterpret metaphor for fact—and send for the doctor to "cure" the "illness." It is as if a television viewer were to send for a television repairman because he

dislikes the program he sees on the screen [in a note to the text, see Szasz, 1973]. (Szasz, 1961, 2nd ed. 1974, pp. x–xi)

Mental illness is a metaphor and a question that needs to be asked is whether the distinction as commonly practiced between conscious and unconscious thought, between "immaterial" (in reality "material") life and the body is not too sharp and overdetermined.

Moreover, most interesting is the problem Szasz raises when he claims that we must shift our attention from the individual to the relation. The individual does not flourish separately from other individuals, but is part of a network of relationships. To reach some form of understanding *à propos* the expressive potential of the relation to the other, context must be foregrounded, the relation itself, exteriority, which no doubt is interiorized, but in any case the relation must be taken into account. This is a pivotal issue investing the question of identity, but with a shift in focus from the individual—conceived as a delineated and determined entity, individual in the sense of "not divided," integral, compact, therefore easily identifiable—to the relation, thereby developing an approach to subjectivity that is typical of semiotics (Petrilli, 2013; Ponzio, 1996, 2006b).

All this entails the problem of the complex relation between the so-called interpreted sign and the interpretant sign, between one sign and another sign that interprets the former, where the interpretant/interpreting sign may be another voice of my own self, the other among the many voices constitutive of self, as much as the voice or voices of the other beyond my own self, beyond my own body, the voice of the other external to self, in a dialogue that is open-ended and ongoing (Petrilli, 2010; Sebeok, Petrilli, & Ponzio, 2001).

The Dialogic Nature of the Self

Szasz is well read in linguistics and philosophy of language. In *The Meaning of Mind* he criticizes linguistics and the neurosciences for reducing the concept of mind to a set of brain functions, a trend he describes as biologistic and oversimplifying. From this point of view he takes issue with the preeminent philosopher of language John R. Searle for establishing a cause and effect relationship between brain and consciousness: "Searle makes consciousness (minding) an attribute of brain, not persons," and treats "mind and brain as if they were the same thing, referring to 'it' as the 'mind/brain'" (Szasz, 1996, p. 82; see also Petrilli and Ponzio, 2016, pp. 128–132).

For his part, Szasz describes the relation between unconscious and conscious, inner and outer, "immaterial" and "material" life, so-called "mind" and "body," and does so in terms of interrupted continuity. Mind, consciousness, and thought processes are made of language, speech, therefore of what he calls "conversations," dialogue, and interpersonal relationships. Echoing the great Russian philosopher and theoretician of dialogue Mikhail Bakhtin, Szasz proposes a "dialogic" conception of psychic life: the mind is made of voices, of what he calls "self-conversations," not only with the outer other with respect to one's own self, but with the inner other, not only with the other *from* self, but with the other *of* self. It ensues that thought processes converge with the capacity for dialogue, which, in turn, entails the capacity for listening (Petrilli, 2007). Like Bakhtin, Szasz, too, praises the capacity to hear voices, internal voices as much as external voices (see Petrilli "Man, Word and the Other," in Thellefsen & Sorensen, ed. 2014, pp. 5–12). Consciousness consists of a multiplicity of voices in dialogue with each other, internally to the same consciousness as much as externally with the voices of the other beyond self.

In chapter 1 of *The Meaning of Mind*, titled "Language: Self-conversation," Szasz cites Bakhtin from *The Dialogic Imagination* (the 1981 English translation of the 1975 Russian original, *Voprosy literatury i estetiki*). Bakhtin thematizes thought and speech in terms of the "speaking person" and his discourse. With reference to the sphere of ethical and legal thought and discourse, for example, all fundamental categories of enquiry and evaluation refer to speaking persons as such: "conscience," that is, the "voice of conscience," the "inner word"; "repentance," that is, a "free admission," a "statement of wrongdoing by the person himself"; "truth and falsehood"; "being liable and not liable," and so forth (Petrilli, 2012b; Ponzio, 2006a, 2015).

Moreover, Szasz cites the following passage by Bakhtin, "An independent, responsible and active discourse is *the* fundamental indicator of an ethical, legal and political human being" (Bakhtin, 1981, pp. 349–350), in support of his own conception of the subject as a "moral agent." According to Szasz, in fact, to assume responsibility for one's own voice is a characteristic of human agency (Szasz, 1996, p. 12). However, his vision of "moral agency" as predicated of the subject calls for questioning, as illustrated by Augusto Ponzio in the third part of the present text.

In any case we cannot but undersign Szasz's dialogic conception of what he calls "self-conversation," that is, talking to oneself, believing, conjecturing, considering, contemplating, debating, deliberating, meditating, musing, pondering, presuming, reasoning, reflecting, ruminating, supposing, surmising, and, of course, thinking (see Petrilli, 2013, pp. xix–xxvii, and the relative Foreword by Ponzio). All such activities are considered as proof of the dialogic nature of consciousness and human relations. Verbal speech acts cannot be reduced to the intentional exchange of rejoinders among speakers; that is, to what Bakhtin calls "formal dialogue" as distinct from so-called "substantial dialogue" (Ponzio, 2006, 2014). Speech acts are both inner and outer and always diaologic. In the words of Szasz:

"Recognizing the ubiquity of self-conversation is an indispensable antidote against the currently conventional view that regards (normal) speech as a verbal act that one person directs to another person or persons [. . .]; and that classifies some inner dialogues as normal (meditating, reflecting), and others as abnormal (hearing voices, being plagued by invasive thoughts)" (Szasz, 1996, p. 13).

To further illustrate the dialogic conception of speech and its significance for human consciousness, Szasz cites Bakhtin yet again, this time from his 1986 collection, *Speech Genres & Other Late Essays* (the English translation of the posthumous original Russian 1979 collection, *Estetika slovesnogo tvorchestva*). Listening is described by Bakhtin as involving an active, responsive attitude. In a relation of understanding, what we recognize as "responsive understanding," "participative understanding," the listener responds to the meaning of an utterance, whether to agree or disagree with it, enhance it, question it, and so forth. In live speech, understanding is responsive, indeed it elicits a responsive attitude, so that, in Bakhtin's words "the listener becomes the speaker" (1986, p. 68), as Szasz also evidences.

In fact, according to the latter's interpretation of Bakhtin, understanding the other implies the capacity to respond to the other, to assume a responsive attitude toward the other. And a "responsive" attitude also implies a "responsible" attitude toward the other, one which is only possible on the basis of listening: "because we love, like, or respect him, or want him to love, like, or respect us. People who are fond of each other often say, 'We understand each other'" (Szasz, 1996, pp. 20, 25–26; see also Ponzio, Petrilli, & Ponzio, 2005). Conversely, the failure to understand the other is often connected with the failure to listen to him. The "unsympathetic listener becomes the uncomprehending hearer," indicating a lack of understanding which Szasz believes characterizes the relationship between the psychiatrist and his psychotic patient when the latter is diagnosed by the former as "crazy" and/or unintelligible, the result of some mental disease. On his part, when practicing psychotherapy, Szasz does not present himself as a "professional of mental health." On the contrary, the difficult task he sets himself is to enter into "conversation" with the other and listen to him in his singularity.

Writing and the Body

Szasz does not use the term "dialogized" which we borrow from Bakhtin. Underlining the plurilinguistic, multiaccentuated, polylogic nature of identity, Bakhtin thematized "dialogized plurilingualism" wherein languages encounter each other and mutually interpret each other. The reference is to "internal plurilingualism" as much as to "external plurilingualism," whether we are speaking about language or subjectivity. Identity is not something compact. In the heart of identity there is otherness, and with otherness many voices, a situation that Virginia Woolf's literary writing evidences very clearly, together with her own life with all its contradictions. Szasz draws our attention, for example, to the contradiction between Virginia, author of *Mrs. Dalloway*, who is critical of psychiatrists, and Virginia, who in real-life circumstances submits to psychiatric therapy. But this too is a performance, a representation of the contradictions that inevitably pervade life, existence, and relations with oneself as much as with others.

Szasz develops a critique of the myth of "mental illness," but also, more generally, of the grammar of everyday life, of the world-as-it-is, of life in its articulation into roles based on the logic of closed identity. The logic of identity is functional to the constitution of affiliations, aggregations, of abstract concepts, of roles connected with sex, class, religion, and race, among others, and is always ready to sacrifice the other, to expunge the other (on this account see the writings of another preeminent American philosopher and semiotician, Charles Morris, in particular his book of 1948, *The Open Self*). Szasz not only criticizes psychiatry with its vocation for surveyance and social *control*, but also the commonplaces of psychiatric discourse when it does not focus sufficiently on the problem of encounter with the other, on listening, and hospitality—in Bakhtinian terms "dialogical listening" and "participative interaction" with the word of the other, hospitality toward the other structural to the self and its manifold voices.

Throughout the whole course—theoretical and practical—of his career, Szasz tends toward listening to the other, "listening" that is altogether different from institutional "wanting to hear," demanding to know how things stand. Listening is the propensity for opening toward the other before and beyond roles and identities, for hospitality toward the situation of multivoicedness, whether internal or external to the same speaker, to the same consciousness. Listening is the necessary condition for speaking and for hospitality toward the single individual's uniqueness and singularity. What Szasz calls "madness" is also the refusal to put the various parts of self, the various voices of self, into communication with each other, refusal to allow the self's multiple selves to dialogue with each other. Rather than search for the condition of listening and hospitality toward one's own differences, toward the various spheres of one's own life, these differences are kept distinct and separate from each other; their languages are stopped from entering into relations of "dialogized plurilingualism," as Bakhtin would say.

For what concerns the importance Szasz attached to encounter and listening, while he was radically critical of psychiatry, he recognized that psychoanalysis, if practiced correctly, could take the form of a confidential conversation and help people deal better with their problems. However, in contrast with Freud, psychoanalysis most often is not practiced in these terms, neither in the United States, nor in Europe: the psychoanalyst as well is a physician free to drug and hospitalize a patient. Despite a nonmedical psychoanalytic tradition as represented by such personalities as Anna Freud, Melanie Klein, Erik Erikson, Erich Fromm, Bruno Bettelheim, Robert Waelder, psychoanalysis in the United States is considered a medical activity close to psychiatry.

Once he had graduated in medicine and begun practicing psychiatry, Szasz soon learnt that to be wrong could be dangerous, but to be right in a society where that which is false is thought to be right by the majority can be even more fatal. In the past false truths structural to the system of beliefs of a whole society were generally of the religious order, currently they are also of the political and medical orders.

Unlike illnesses of the body in which case we search for causes and cures, the concept of "mental illness" is a myth and concerns behavioral patterns. Szasz distinguishes between sickness and behavior and maintains that one of the limits of psychiatric language consists of applying metaphorical figures drawn from the vocabulary of disease to behavior. Deviated behaviors varying from the merely eccentric to the criminal are discriminated simply on the basis of confusing descriptions of bodily disease with evaluations of the moral, ethical, ideological, and political orders.

When practicing psychotherapy, Szasz, as anticipated above, does not present himself as a health professional, but installs a "conversation" with the other in order to listen to his problems.

À propos of his conceptualization of "deviation" in relation to his case study on Virginia Woolf, Szasz makes an interesting distinction between "deviation up" and "deviation down," which, in response to my query and in line with his design to use "straightforward English prose," rather than medical terminology (unless he is discussing medical issues), he clarified to me in the following terms: "'Deviation,' formerly a sociological term, has become part of the American language. Deviation—departure from the norm, average. Genius—too smart, gifted = up. Mad—too troublesome, dependent = down" (Szasz to Petrilli, e-mail 11 June, 2008).

Szasz belongs to a tradition of thought that is connected with classical liberalism and is influenced by such figures from the past as Thomas Jefferson, John Stuart Mill, and Ludwig von Mises. Consequently, he believes that religion and state, medicine and state, psychiatry and state should be kept separate. What Szasz does not accept is coercion and the medicalization of society. Nobody should be forced to consult with a psychiatrist, to be hospitalized, or take drugs just as nobody should be forced to believe in a system of ideas. Szasz opposes coercion, the exercise of power and dominion over the will of the single individual, which he described as a form of abuse commonly practiced in the name of science.

In the social-political sphere, Szasz engaged on various fronts. He struggled against the classification of homosexuality as an illness, against prohibition concerning the use of drugs, against the various forms of sexual therapy, which he considered as forms of prostitution and pornography masquerading as "education for mental health." A firm point for Szasz, personal beliefs aside, was that the state should not interfere with questions of the moral order. Moreover, while he defended the right to suicide, he opposed the idea that suicide should be assisted by the physician. He considered such a practice as yet another form of abuse given that in consonance with the medicalization of the social, it endorses the physician with the power to control the life of others to the point even of collaborating in the freedom to die.

By now famous worldwide for his critical vision of psychiatric and psychoanalytic practice, Szasz continued opposing coercion by psychiatry and its justifications for the whole time of his confrontational career, thereby continuing the struggle initiated from the very beginning. On this account, particularly significant are the title of his books *Coercion as Cure: A Critical History of Psychiatry*, 2007, *Psychiatry: The Science of Lies*, 2008, and *Antipsychiatry: Quackery Squared*, 2009.

Szasz introduced the expression "therapeutic state" to indicate the political power of physicians, in particular the psychiatrist's. As an agent of the therapeutic state the psychiatrist is authorized to deprive an individual of his freedom, if judged to be a "threat to himself and to others." Szasz never accepted the fact that a psychiatrist could replace the law, deciding on the nonimputability of a crime on the basis of the condition of "mental health" or "mental illness" of the defendant. Moreover, he believes that the state has a right to intervene on issues that concern public health, for example, stopping a person with an infectious disease from circulating freely, but not to interfere with private affairs as in the case of drug use. Good/evil, good/bad, safe/dangerous, and risky/not risky do not describe the quality of a drug, but, if anything, are paradigms relating to its use, which does not concern the state but is a question of the ethical order.

Yet again in his book on Virginia Woolf, Szasz develops his caustic critique of psychiatry and of the "myth of mental illness" through a detailed and unbiased reconstruction of her life. He reveals a great capacity for listening in contrast to dominant discourse on the "mad genius," that is, on the relationship between mental illness and artistic talent ("deviation up"), whether in literary criticism, philosophy, the human sciences generally or in common language.

The approach to Virginia Woolf's madness and suicide in this book may be described as transdisciplinary more than interdisciplinary, involving various disciplines including psychiatry, medicine, law, ethics, but also literary criticism, philosophy, linguistics, women's studies, cultural studies, and above all writing, literary writing.

Fundamentally Szasz critiques the absurdities of "psychopathology." However, he also demolishes that paper world which "culture" erects by superimposing a mythological subject, obtained with a *chiaroscuro* effect (good/bad, healthy/sick, capable/incapable, integrated/misfitted), over the singularity, uniqueness, incomparability of every single life in itself. This is not only a question of the myth of "mental illness," generally considered as "somebody else's affair," but rather it also involves sexual identity, affiliation, civil status, functionality, identification, roles, profession, in brief, one's "place in the world" and this concerns each one of us, whether "a genius" or "not a genius," "normal" or "abnormal." Called to issue is not only the psychiatric vision and its application as a form of social control; but also the commonplaces characteristic of psychiatric discourse that do not necessarily favor encounter as offered by Szasz with an unknown and unlistened to Virginia Woolf. Refractory to separation among discourse genres, this book escapes the boundaries of the essay genre and follows the dynamics of a narration.

In this study on Virginia's madness and marriage, "*My Madness Saved Me*," Szasz presents a critical reflection on human relationships, which inevitably pass through the word, are constructed in the word, the narrated word. Szasz listens to Virginia Woolf, the writer and the woman, as much as to the characters she invents and her entire real-life entourage. He evokes their words and reflects on them, drawing on Virginia's literary writing, her novels and short stories, as much as on her nonliterary writing, her letters, diaries, but without neglecting what her biographers have to say, as much as the medicine-men, the witch-doctors of psychiatry and psychiatrized psychoanalysis, her denigrators, and again her admirers and emulators, literary critics and feminists all. Inevitably, Szasz clashes with the pretensions of those who claim to know, judge, classify, absolve or condemn, especially on the part of those whom Szasz unmasks as amateurs and tricksters (under this aspect, particularly interesting are the texts in the appendix to this book on Virginia, where in no uncertain terms he openly criticizes the charlatans of psychiatry and psychoanalysis).

Language Matters

Szasz often reflects on the meaning of words connected with the problems he deals with: sickness, disease, medicine, humanity, freedom, responsibility, power, control, psychiatry, body, mind, mental illness; and on the relationship between these words and their referents in different languages. In English up until the seventeenth century, the word *mind* did not exist as a noun, only the verb *to mind* and *minding*: to concern oneself with, to take an interest in, to care for, to guard, to look after, to take care of, to pay attention, to heed, to beware, to attend to, to watch over, and so forth. In the paper he delivered at the 2003 congress at the Villa Borromeo, "Why I wrote *The Myth of Mental Illness*," Szasz explains that: "The Freudian unconscious has nothing to do with *mind*. [. . .] from a scientific point of view mind does not exist more than the soul does [. . .] What is study of the mind? If the mind does not exist, how does it get sick? *Quod erat demonstrandum*. End of story. [. . .] I have been defining this as the therapeutic state for over forty years now. Once upon a time there existed theological states,

37

their legitimation and functioning were safeguarded by the idea of God, religion and the Bible. Today this is gradually replaced by medical criteria, [. . .] indeed prevalently by so-called psychiatric criteria" (Szasz, in *Medicina e umanità*, p. 20). Szasz confirms his rejection of coercion toward the so-called "mentally ill," of the use of psychotropic drugs, electroshock, forced hospitalization, and repeats that he does not recognize the condition of mental illness: "All my work revolves around the observation that mental illness does not exist, just as witchcraft does not exist. Just as the unicorn does not exist. In other words, it is not possible to demonstrate the mental health of a person, because it is not possible to demonstrate mental illness" (Ibid., pp. 32–33).

In reply to my question whether there was a reason why in his book on Virginia Woolf's madness he never used the term "psychopathology" (e-mail 1 January, 2008), Szasz offered the following explanation: "the term 'psychopathology' confers an air of medical legitimacy to the phenomenon which, on the contrary, is altogether absent from the expression 'mental illness'—which is vague and almost void, deprived of any sense. In all my writings I avoid medical terms (or terms that resound in a medical sense), unless of course I am referring to real sicknesses." And, in fact, in a subsequent e-mail exchange, dated 10 January, 2008, he repeated that "Yes, indeed. This is the whole point of the book, that Virginia Woolf was not a 'sick,' 'crazy' woman; she was a proud, independent *person*." Indeed in the same letter he suggested that "Perhaps, to underscore this, you should add a 'Translator's note' to alert the reader that the language choice is very important, subtly communicative. (You are *of course* the ideal translator as you know me, my work, etc.)."

In relation to Szasz's attention for language matters, most interesting are his comments on the appropriate pronoun to use in discourse wherein the opposition male/female is not the issue. In reply to my observations about the use of terms like "*uomo*" in Italian and "man" in English with the general meaning of "*antropos*," therefore not in opposition to "*gynè*," Szasz stated that "1. The he/she format is a bad joke. Can you imagine Shakespeare doing that? Political correctness in the very worst sense. 2. Writing always 'she'—which is an alternative many American writers now adopt—is *no less* sexist. Just the opposite. 3. *Hungarian*. Are you aware that Hungarian is a totally genderless language! (Gender etc. must be inferred from the context, situation.) And of course Hungarian culture was/is not less sexist than other languages and other cultures" (Szasz to Petrilli, e-mail 10 gennaio, 2008).

In our exchanges on the relation between sign and language studies and psychiatry, Szasz observed that "my basic work—especially in *Pain and Pleasure* and *The Myth of Mental Illness*—belongs, properly speaking, to logic, rhetoric, and semiotics, not medicine or psychiatry" (Szasz to Petrilli, June 7, 2011). However, he pointed out what he described as a lack of mutual interest between "linguists" and "psychiatrists." As he wrote in another message: "Show me one linguist (other than Korzybski) who addressed psychiatry" (October 6, 2011). In another series of exchanges, I observed that "there exist areas of research like psycholinguistics and psychosemiotics which put together studies on language and studies in psychology, psychiatry, etc. Frederik van Eeden, poet, writer, philosopher psychiatrist acted as a bridge between Victoria Welby [. . .] and the Significs Movement in the Netherlands, which involved psychiatrists working on language and communication (first half of the twentieth century) [. . .]. Charles Morris wrote a book called *The Open Self*, and Peirce's sign theory is also closely connected to subject theory. But what about Julia Kristeva? A psychiatrist, psychoanalyst, and semiotician by profession, but also Jacques Lacan, or Armando Verdiglione thanks to whom we met?" (Petrilli to Szasz, e-mail October 7, 2011). To this Szasz commented: "Yes, I know. But psychiatrists have power over people, they can and do deprive them of liberty. To me it matters little what they say about their work. What they do is what matters. Semioticians, like historians or mathematicians, have no such power. I am sending you a chapter that discusses Lacan and psychiatric power [To his e-mail Tom attached chapter 6, 'Antipsychiatry Abroad: Psychiatry Redux,' from his 2009 book *Antipsychiatry: Quackery Squared*, Syracuse Press] . . ." (Szasz to Petrilli, e-mail October 7, 2011).

Whatever our considerations regarding his interpretation of Virginia Woolf's life and works, the position proposed by Szasz is no doubt worthy of consideration when he claims that the focus must be shifted away from the individual taken in isolation and examined internally, in her "physical-mental structure," with the pretension of formulating classifications and judgments passed off as "scientific." Instead, the focus must be on her relationships, that is, the context of her relationships with others. In this sense, the text (not only Virginia's works, but also her life), demands to be read in context, and the context, as Augusto Ponzio demonstrates in his own text below, can only be traced in the word, in writing, whether public (as in her novels) or private (as in her letters and diaries), in her own word or in the word, the "witness" of others, but in any case always in the word, and not in some place outside it, in the "facts"—as though the facts do not exert, uphold, even establish, and certainly communicate their truths through words.

This is a crucially important point which invests the question of identity and requires a shift of attention from the individual—understood as a pre-established, predefined entity, monological, integral, compact, therefore identifiable and classifiable—to the relationship, to the word, the utterance, to the work of interpreting and reading, to a project, to life with all its problematics of the semiotic order. And such problematics concern above all the relationship between the interpretant sign and interpreted sign, between the sign and the other sign that interprets it, where the interpreting sign can either be another one of my own voices, another one of my many voices, or the voice of another person outside me, the external other. In both cases the situation is one of ongoing, perpetual dialogue.

Reading Virginia's Word with Him—Augusto Ponzio

In *Psychopathology of Everyday Life*, Freud's fundamental thesis is that the behavior of people considered to be mentally abnormal is "governed" by the same principles that govern the behavior of people considered as mentally normal. Once this was recognized, Freud could choose between two pathways. Either conclude that there is no such thing as mental illness, and therefore write books on the normality of mentally ill people. Or, conclude, as he did, that the healthy minded are like sick people, and write about the abnormality of the healthy minded. He in fact coined the expression "pathology of everyday life" insinuating, successfully, that normal behavior is similar to abnormal behavior, and that within certain limits each one of us is mentally ill. As we know, this standpoint became the basis of modern psychiatry.

—Thomas S. Szasz, "Prefazione alla nuova edizione italiana" [Preface to the new Italian edition], *The Myth of Mental Illness* 1961

The Context Is in the Text

It is important to read a text remaining in the text, looking for meaning in the text and not in the context external to it. In an essay of 1981, "Il contesto nel testo" (The context in the text), the Italian critic Arcangelo Leone de Castris maintained that we must not abandon the text, as instead literary criticism often does, to look in the author's private life for elements in support of an interpretation, or in his relations of the ideological and political orders. The context is in the text itself, in the word, in writing.

However, this is not the way we usually proceed. The vice alluded to can be expressed in terms of a notion analyzed by Sergio Dalla Val in his paper, "La materia del dire e del fare" (The material of saying and doing, 2011): "the subject."

Subjectus, "that which lies underneath," "that which supports."

If we assume the existence of a subject, what can occur in our case is that instead of discussing Virginia Woolf's writing, we focus on the substratum that supports it, the underlying structure. But this is a subtantialist, ontological, and metaphysical view we must get free of.

Thomas Szasz invites us to do exactly this, making an important contribution in this sense with his book, "My Madness Saved Me": The Madness and Marriage of Virginia Woolf.

But to what point? The title "My Madness Saved Me" is an "utterance" and certainly not a "sentence," as the linguists would say. The utterance tells of the possibility of "writing." But "writing" here is not understood in the sense of transcription, graphic signs traced on a surface, as they teach us at school (the birth of writing and transition from prehistory to history!); our reference is to writing as "construction," thanks to which Virginia Woolf went on her journey, and invented a new world, a life.

About the Moral Agent Virginia

To believe that Virginia was acting and that she deliberately recited the part of a mad woman, as Szasz insinuates (indeed, aims to demonstrate), means to believe that we have a subject, on one hand, and actions, thoughts, words, writing based on that subject, on the other.

This is the fallacy of the foundations, of the substratum, the subject, precisely, and of the "accidents" that "stand" on the subject. This is the ontological fallacy which is part of the places of discourse. It leads us to believe that we must always "search underneath," in the depths, that we must excavate, discover. On the contrary, that which is hidden and cannot be seen is always on the surface, in the text, "the context is in the text," in writing, in the word, in the letter, before our very eyes, as Edgar A. Poe says with his tale about the "purloined letter." Unlike the Prefect, the Police Commissar, Auguste Dupin knew where to look because he knew that the Minister who had stolen the letter was not only a mathematician, but also a poet. And as a poet, a writer, there was no doubt that he should have hidden the purloined letter where generally nobody would look for it: that is, on the surface, in full view.

So, how do we read this book by Szasz? As the effort, however partial, to dissipate the heavy prejudice that there exists a carrying subject, a *facteur*—*Le facteur de la verité* (1975) is the title of a book by Jacques Derrida; *facteur* also means postman, in Italian "portalettere," "letter-carrier"—a carrier, this being a central concept in the "place," the "commonplace" of illness, and for what concerns "our own" discourse of "mental illness." The myth of mental illness is exactly this: to believe that there exists a sick subject on one hand, a carrier of this type of sickness, and that all his actions, on the other, are a consequence of the condition of being sick.

This idea is based on the belief that there exist mechanical cause–effect relationships, but this too is a *forma mentis* we need to get free of: we now know at different levels and from different scientific perspectives that there exist *feedback* mechanisms, where the effect retroacts on the cause. So that—as Hume had already stated—this too is a fallacy: to consider what comes first as the cause of what comes later. Virginia behaved in a certain way, therefore from the very outset "she was made" in a certain way, as a consequence . . . But what is observed as coming first is only retroactively perceived as the cause of what is perceived in a subsequent moment.

Szasz takes a stand against the idea of an illness carrier, in our specific case mental illness, which militates against the "myth of mental illness." Therefore with Szasz the claim is that we are not to search for the cause of what happens in Virginia's life in her "mental illness"—her choices, behavior, geniality as a writer, her suicide: there is no carrier, *no mentally ill* subject at the origin of her actions.

At the same time, however, Szasz does recognize the existence of a carrying subject; the *facteur* does exist, but this is not the mentally ill subject. The subject is there and is the cause, but this subject as thematized by Szasz is a "moral agent," a subject responsible for his own actions, words, writings, a subject that decides, recites, simulates, calculates, chooses what serves him best. The subject, *substratum*, carrier: these concepts from the places of dominant discourse remain in Szasz and his writings. Therefore the search for a unilinear route continues, the search for a thread that draws everything together has not ended. We may speak of a thread, but also of a track, a "unidirectional track" that crosses through the whole of one's life. According to Szasz, all of life is guided, channeled, directed, determined by its "moral agent": "a moral agent who used mental illness, psychiatry and her husband."

Virginia Woolf dissents through writing, precisely: she rejects and withdraws from the subject, from cause, mastery, command, control, identification, unilinear channeling, in historical succession. Writing itself, literary writing is incompatible with the idea of a "moral agent": the writer cannot be a subject. And owing to his expectations as a subject, to his claims to self-management, to mastery, the subject cannot be a writer. He might be a scrivener, yes, but certainly not a writer in the sense of literary writing.

With reference to Virginia Woolf's novel, *To the Lighthouse*: the whole beginning chapter is dedicated to the uncertainty about going or not to the lighthouse and the weather. But when she moves on to the next chapter, there is no trace whatsoever of the preceding situation; nothing more is left of young James's dream place, of that "important question" raised during an evening in September on the eve of the First World War. Things have changed completely, and those who seemed to be the main characters of the fabula, Mrs. Ramsay, her son Andrew and daughter Prue have all passed away—and even when, ten years later, Mr. Ramsay goes on the trip with the children, James, who had desired it so intensely and hoped in good weather, is now another person. Not only: while the text dwells on minor details describing the state of abandonment and degradation of the house (that had merely acted as a backdrop in the first chapter and is now the proscenium, with the curtain unexpectedly closed already), it only reserves less than two lines to narrate the death of mother and her two children.

The Madness of Writing

The subject is one thing and writing—the word, life—is another. Mental illness is one thing. It consists in considering oneself as a subject, as a cause. Madness is another. It belongs to writing, to life, to the voyage.

Thomas Szasz is not aware of this distinction; he does not distinguish madness, craziness thus understood from acting as a truth carrier; and he is not aware of "madness" as the very condition for writing. The omniscient narrator can invent the *fabula*, but he may lack the plot; he knows *what* to say, but not *how* to say it. Woolf is a great writer because she does not aim to master the word, she listens to it; she does not plan a story, she follows it; she writes writing.

Certainly, in her writing there is the woman question, just as in every piece of writing there is the sexual question: not in terms of sexual identity, but of sexual difference, singularity; this is not the question of gender or belonging, of affiliation, attribution, assignment to one group rather than to another on the basis of personal credentials. In Virginia's case the woman question is the question of difference considered in terms of singularity, of corporeality, in its specific space-time. Space-time plays a central role in Virginia Woolf's writing. It presents its own specific characteristics, its own cypher, its own special way of expressing materiality, corporeity—the unsayable: its own special way of expressing each single individual's unreplaceability, each single individual's noninterchangeability with the place of another single individual, with another singularity. Each singularity is endowed with its own materiality, corporeity. This enables us to speak of difference understood as singularity and uniqueness, in relation to which madness is something impossible to catalogue, to classify and explain.

With Virginia Woolf we can say that with respect to the male subject, as is Mr. Ramsay, writing is feminine or is not; in other words, the writer is the person who says nothing in his own name, who takes a listening position. Virginia Woolf succeeds in rendering the multiple voices of a text that is expected to have its own voice. She writes keeping silent, she listens and does not speak in her own name; her characters speak instead. Of course, in the face of a writer who has escaped his own identity, including sexual identity, his own contemporaneity, accomplishing the situation of exotopic distancing, there is always the critic who contradicts him. This critic attempts to reconduct the writer to his assumed place of origin, to those very same places of discourse he had evaded. This is the critic obsessed with searching for the context outside the text, who attempts to explain the text by searching for the subject who caused it.

An aspect of this book by Szasz deserves special attention: that is, when he claims that Virginia Woolf cannot be described as being mentally ill in the same way as she can be described as being English and a woman, or that Leonard can be described as a Jew. This is another instance where ontology reemerges in Szasz despite his critique of mental illness. This again is another instance of the idea of the origin, the substratum, the beginning of the word, of writing, the idea of geneology, the category of being, the subject. Unfortunately, this way of reasoning has deep roots in us all. But every moment in the life of each one of us, on the professional, family, political levels, in "public" life and in the "private," is in the relation with others, in the encounter among words. The idea of identity difference, for example between communitarian and so-called extra-communitarian, between the Jew and the Palestinian, between man and woman, builds a trap which captures us and which we cannot get free of.

Thomas Szasz makes an incredibly courageous effort to destroy this trap. However, he still abides by the idea that there exists a Virginia Woolf as a deciding subject. This is the idea of freedom *over* the word, instead of freedom *of* the word. Instead, the writer is a person who leaves the word free, who takes a listening position, whose aim is no longer to take the word or to give the word, who no longer deludes himself into believing that he is the word's master. As Freud once said: nobody is master in one's own home, the reference being to one's "own" body and above all to one's "own" language.

References

Bakhtin, M. M. (1981). *The dialogic imagination. Four essays.* Edited by C. Emerson and M. Holquist. Austin: University of Texas Press.

Bakhtin, M. M. (1986). *Speech genres & other late essays.* (V. W. McGee, Trans; C. Emerson & M. Holquist, Eds.). Austin: University of Texas Press.

Dalla Val, S. (2011). La material del dire e del fare. *La città del secondo rinascimento, 43,* 9.

Derrida, J. (1975). *Le facteur de la vérité. Poétique,* n. 21; repris dans *La Carte postale, de Socrate à Freud et au-delà.* Paris: Flammarion, 1980, pp. 439–524. It. trans. *Il fattore della verità,* by F. Zambon, Milan, Adelphi, 1978.

Freud, S. (1901). *Psychopathology of everyday life* (The Standard Edition). London: Norton.

Leone de Castris, A. (1981). Il contest nel testo. Per una coscienza storica dello specifico letterario. In C. A. Augieri, F. Pappalardo, A. Ponzio, P. Voza, Postfazione di, & N. Vendola (Eds.), *Nelle forme della scrittura e oltre. Teoria, storia e critica della letteratura,* (pp. 233–263). Lecce: Milella.

Morris, C. (1948). *Open self.* (S. Petrilli, Bari, Graphis, Trans. and Intro.). New York: Prentice Hall.

Petrilli, S. (2003). Semioetica e salute della vita. In *Stress. La clinica della vita. Il secondo rinascimento. Logica e industria della parola. Cultura, arte, impresa, politica, finanza, comunicazione.* Atti del Congresso Internazionale, 10–12 May 2002, 3–5 March, pp. 119–23, 125–30. Milan: Spirali/Vel.

Petrilli, S. (Ed.). (2007). *Philosophy of language as the art of listening: On Augusto Ponzio's scientific research.* Bari: Edizioni dal Sud.

Petrilli, S. (2009). Follia e psichiatria. La critica di Thomas Szasz al mito della malattia mentale. [Introduction to Thomas Szasz *La mia follia mi ha salvato.*] *La follia e il matrimonio di Virginia Woolf* (S. Petrilli, Ed. and It. Trans.). 7–59. Milan: Spirali. [= It. Trans. of T. Szasz 2006].

Petrilli, S. (2012a). *Expression and interpretation in language.* New Brunswick, U.S.A. and London: Transaction Publishers.

Petrilli, S. (2012b). *Alrove e altrimenti. Filosofia del linguaggio, critica letteraria e teoria della traduzione in, con e a partire da Bachtin.* Milan: Mimesis.

Petrilli, S. (2013). *The self as a sign, the world, and the other. Living semiotics*, with a foreword by Augusto Ponzio, xii–xv. New Brunswick (USA) and London: Transaction Publishers.

Petrilli, S. (2014). *Sign systems and semioethics. Communication, translation and values*. Berlin and New York: De Gruyter Mouton.

Petrilli, S. (ed.) (2014). *Semioetica e comunicazione globale* (*Athanor. Semiotica, Filosofia, Arte, Letteratura, XXIV,17*). Milan: Mimesis.

Petrilli, S., & A. Ponzio. (2016). *Lineamenti di semiotica e di filosofia del linguaggio*. Perugia: Guerra edizioni.

Poe, E. A. (1845). *The purloined letter*. In E. A. Poe *Great tales and poems*. New York: Washington Square Press.

Ponzio, A. (2006a). *The dialogic nature of sign*. Ottawa: Legas.

Ponzio, A. (2006b). *The I questioned: Emmanuel Levinas and the critique of occidental reason*. Special issue of *Subject matter. A journal of communications and the self*, 3, 3.

Ponzio, A. (2007). *A mente. Formazione linguistica e processi cognitivi*. Perugia: Guerra Edizioni.

Ponzio, A. (2011). *In altre parole*. Milano: Mimesis.

Ponzio, A. (2013). *Fuori luogo. L'esorbitante nella produzione dell'identico*. Milan: Mimesis.

Ponzio, A. (Ed.). (2014). Bachtin e il suo circolo. *Opere 1919–1930*, bilingual Russian/Italian text (A. Ponzio, It. Trans., Intro. and Comment) with the assistance of L. Ponzio ("Il pensiero occidentale," directed by G. Reale). Milan: Bompiani.

Ponzio, A. (2015). *Tra semiotica e letteratura. Introduzione a Michail Bachtin*. Milan: Bompiani.

Ponzio, A., Petrilli, S., & Ponzio, J. (2005). *Reasoning with Levinas*. Ottawa: Legas.

Schaler, J. A. (Ed. and Introduction). (2004). *Szasz under fire: The psychiatric abolitionist faces his critics* (A. Jeffrey, Ed.). Schaler. Chicago and La Salle, IL: Open Court.

Szasz, T. S. (1957). *Pain and pleasure. A study of bodily feelings*. (New ed. 1988). New York: Basic Books: Syracuse University Press.

Szasz, T. S. (1961). *The myth of mental illness. Foundations of a theory of personal conduct*. (Revised edition, 1974; New Italian translation, *Il mito della matattia mentale*, by Francesco Saba Sardi, Milan, Spirali, 2003). New York: Perennial/HarperCollins.

Szasz, T. S. (1973). Mental illness as a metaphor, *Nature*, 242, 305.

Szasz, T. S. (1978a). *The myth of psychotherapy: Mental healing as religion, rhetoric, and repression*. (New Edition Syracuse University Press, Syracuse, 1988; trad. it. *Il mito della psicoterapia*, Feltrinelli, Milano, 1981). Garden City, New York: Doubleday Anchor.

Szasz, T. S. (1978b). Una follia legale. La dissidenza. La psichiatria in Russia e negli Stati Uniti. *Lo Stato. Giornale internazionale di cultura*, n. 1, Spirali: Milan.

Szasz, T. S. (1984). *The therapeutic state: Psychiatry in the mirror of current events*. Buffalo, New York: Prometheus Books.

Szasz, T. S. (1990). L'incapace. Lo specchio morale del conformismo. (It. Trans. by C. Frua De Angeli). Milan: Spirali/Vel.

Szasz, T. S. (1996). The meaning of mind. Language, morality and neuroscience. Westport, CT: Praeger Publisher.

Szasz, T. S. (2000). La battaglia per la salute. (It. Trans. A. Guerra, A. Spadafora, L. Zanardi). Milan: Spirali.

Szasz, T. S. (2002). Straight talk about suicide. Freeman. Ideas on Liberty; It. Trans. "Se vogliamo parlare senza infingimenti del suicidio," by S. Petrilli, Corposcritto, 4, 137–140.

Szasz, T. S. (2004a). Perché ho scritto 'Il mito della malattia mentale. In Medicina e umanità. Atti del congresso internazionale. Milan: Spirali.

Szasz, T. S. (2004b). Protolinguaggio, il linguaggio del corpo. It. Trans. by S. Petrilli, PLAT, Quaderni del dipartimento di Pratiche linguistiche e Analisi di Testi, 3, 9–24.

Szasz, T. S. (2006). "My madness saved me." The madness and marriage of Virginia Woolf. New Brunswick (U.S.A.), Transaction Publishers. It. Trans., "La mia follia mi ha salvato." La follia e il matrimonio di Virginia Woolf, ed. and intro., "Follia e psichiatria. La critica di Thomas Szasz al mito della malattia mentale," pp. 7–59, by S. Petrilli, Milan, Spirali.

Szasz, T. S. (2007). Coercion as cure: A critical history of psychiatry. New Brunswick, NJ: Transaction.

Szasz, T. S. (2008). Psychiatry: The science of lies. Syracuse, NY: Syracuse University Press.

Szasz, T. S. (2009). Antipsychiatry: Quackery squared. Syracuse, NY: Syracuse University Press.

Thellefsen, T., & Sorensen, B. (2014). (eds. and Foreword, pp. v–vii). Charles Sanders Peirce in his own words. 100 years of semiotics, communication, and cognition. In Paul C. & Kalevi K. (Eds.). Semiotics, Communication and Cognition (volume 14). Preface by C. de Waal, pp. viii–xv. Berlin and New York: De Gruyter Mouton.

Woolf, V. (1925). Mrs. Dalloway. London: Hogarth Press.

Woolf, V. (1927). To the lighthouse. London: Hogarth Press.

3

What Thomas S. Szasz Has Wrought: A Mixed Assessment

Richard E. Vatz

This writer was a friend and admirer and even a one-time coauthor with Thomas Szasz, perhaps the most consequential iconoclast of the seminal medical pretensions of psychiatry and, to a large extent, psychology as well (Vatz et al., 1985). He was also a major practitioner of rhetorical study, my academic field (Vatz & Weinberg, 1994). Also, Szasz's rhetorical understanding is evident in the latest version of his major work, *The Myth of Mental Illness* (Szasz, 2010).

Szasz's dozens of books and thousands of articles all stemmed from the profundity of his arguments that mental illness is a myth; that is, the mind is not an organ; moreover, the mind does not exist; it is a cognitive construct and therefore cannot be diseased. The brain is, as Szasz pointed out repeatedly, quite obviously a biological organ and thus can be diseased. The use of medical metaphors to characterize people's aberrant behavior has never led to an increased understanding of those behaviors or pathological referents; it merely mystified observers and justified excusing bad or illicit actions and exculpating the perpetrators of such behavior. The apotheosis of such transforming of public acceptance of otherwise unacceptable behavior is the psychological mitigation of destructive or illegal behaviors and especially the insanity plea, through which even murderers can find refuge from incarceration through their being remanded to psychiatric care for a time before eventual release when they are "cured" or in "remission."

Szasz and Mental Illness as Myth and Metaphor

The focus of this chapter is to give a general assessment of whether there is, as a consequence of Szasz's work, a rejection or even a reconsideration by the public or intelligentsia of the rhetorical status of "mental illness" as a medical concept which explains why people do what they do. The Szaszian argument is that establishment or institutional psychiatry "explains" everything while actually labeling without explaining anything. There is no way to empirically make this judgment of the general acceptance of Szasz's negation of "mental illness," and we must rely on anecdotal impressions. The verdict is not by any means an overwhelmingly positive judgment.

The rhetorical refuge of attributing unusually horrible acts or simply unusual actions to mental illness has not noticeably abated since Szasz first questioned the existence of "mental illness" over a half century ago. His thesis has always been clear to the discerning mind, that the term "mental illness" is a metaphor, and, like all metaphors, it cannot be taken literally. To take it literally means that strange and self-defeating behavior should be treated by doctors of the mind and that people are not responsible for their "ill" behavior.

In mid-career during the mid-1970s, Szasz wrote a book titled *Schizophrenia: The Sacred Symbol of Psychiatry* (1976) in which he argued that someone, even a doctor, could know everything there is to be known about schizophrenia and yet be wholly ignorant of medicine.

To my way of thinking, this illustrates one of the reasons why selling the myth of mental illness is so difficult. Schizophrenia is a rare and extremely heterogeneous behavioral phenomenon. Psychiatric "experts" believe schizophrenia is a disease, and they have good reason to claim this is so. They earn their living treating people with diseases. They can't earn a living treating metaphorical diseases. However, it is often portrayed by psychiatrists as exemplary of Szasz's thesis that there is no mental illness. Schizophrenia is often applied lazily by many psychiatrists as a catch-all diagnosis.

Szasz and Neurological Illness

It is important to remember that a small percentage of people labeled (diagnosed) as schizophrenic—often cited as 1 percent of the population of people labeled as mentally ill—*are* brain diseased and cognitively incompetent. These people generally show the signs of disease during an autopsy. A putative or theorized physiological or histological basis for the majority of behaviors diagnosed as mental illness cannot

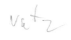
be identified or found during an autopsy, or by searching for signs of depression and anxiety, for example. Signs refer to physical anatomical changes or cellular lesions.

I once asked Dr. Szasz why he didn't concede that schizophrenia could refer to neurological illness, and in conversation he sometimes did in just this sense. He responded to me, and this is not a precise quote but it is close, "Rick, as soon as I concede that schizophrenia can be a neurological disease, you will see an explosion of the diagnoses of schizophrenia. The fact is, of course, that there are neurological diseases, but there is nothing in the diagnostic criteria of schizophrenia that prevents any psychiatrist, psychologist or social worker from diagnosing any very seriously problematic person as 'schizophrenic.'" Diagnoses based on symptoms or complaints have to do with clinical medicine. Diagnoses based on signs or objective symptoms and lesions have to do with scientific medicine. How a person feels or doesn't feel is irrelevant to scientific medicine. While symptoms may certainly lead scientists to signs, the majority of diseases are diagnosed through signs, not through symptoms alone. And, as Szasz often pointed out, in no genuine disease is the symptom itself a disease. Indeed, many diseases are asymptomatic, especially in the early stages.

No doubt many people who speak what psychiatrists call unintelligible "word salad" may have a brain disease, but psychiatrists and others who insist that such people are representative of the class of "mentally ill" people are taking advantage of a population that should be seen as brain diseased and *not* mentally ill, rhetorically speaking. Conversely, those who recognize that mental illness is but a metaphor should stop claiming that all schizophrenia is freely chosen behavior, a position that I know from private conversations with Szasz that he didn't believe.

Regardless, Szasz believed that to explicitly concede the point was to allow people to falsely infer that he thought there were some people who were genuinely "mentally ill."

Szasz used to write particularly derisively of those who would argue only that mental illness was overdiagnosed: that mental illness was a major problem, just not as widespread as most people thought. This also called into question the exceedingly low reliability and validity of psychiatric categories, classification, and agreement among diagnosticians and treatments implemented based on their analyses. This was a crucial, yet not a well-known issue for Szasz. The expansion of the estimate of the incidence of mental illness by the psychiatric community, as articulated in major peer-reviewed publications, was no less than prodigious. From the estimates pronounced decades ago that mental illness struck about 10 percent of citizens, calculations and reliability have steadily gone up—including people who drink too much or take too many drugs—to over 50 percent including over 50 percent for college students in one year (Blanco et al., 2008).

In my opinion, Szasz should have allowed publicly, as he did privately, that the mind—a metaphysical construct—could not be ill, but that some people diagnosed with schizophrenia really had brain disease. For example, when the spirochete bacteria for syphilis was discovered in the 1900s, researchers soon realized that many of the people forcibly put into mental hospitals were in fact suffering from the tertiary phase of syphilis, also known as general paresis. This strengthened the belief that people exhibiting abnormal behavior must all have some form physical disease that caused them to be mad. Again, repeatedly, psychiatry, in arguing the existence of mental illness, uses schizophrenia as its "sacred symbol," as Szasz termed it, implicitly representative of all mental illnesses. But it isn't.

Only a negligible number of people are going to see the cognitively bizarre and non-self-serving behaviors of many schizophrenics and say there is "nothing wrong" with that person neurologically. But if critics of psychiatry insist that such people are neurologically sound moral agents, the entire rhetorical battle and maybe the entire rhetorical war will be lost without a change in interpretation of schizophrenic behavior, its meaning and consequences. This does not mean, of course, that the validity of Szasz's argument regarding the nonexistence of mental illness would be undermined if some behavior labeled as schizophrenia is seen as a brain disease. A key point here is how schizophrenia the putative disease is differentiated from schizophrenia the metaphorical disease. In both cases signs do not exist. And symptoms or complaints are an unreliable way of determining the presence of a disease. Sharp pain in the area of one's diaphragm could mean a hiatal hernia, ulcerative colitis, myocardial infarction, appendicitis, pancreatic cancer, or a factitious disease, that is, an indication of patient malingering, fabricated by a person in order to get out of some responsibility. But as Szasz repeatedly pointed out, thoughts and behaviors are not medical symptoms.

The Unpersuasiveness of the Myth of Mental Illness to Virtually Everyone

What measures can one use to ascertain the general public's receptivity to Szasz's argument that mental illness is but a metaphor, explaining nothing concerning the causes or cures or responsibility of aberrant behavior or beliefs? People want to make sense of atrocities that are unpreventable, such as the murders in Roseburg, Oregon, in 2015, wherein a gunman asked victims if they were Christian and shot those who answered in the affirmative. People abhor a vacuum when it comes to trying to understand and predict terrifying behavior in others.

The use of the mystifying rhetoric of mental illness ebbs and flows according to whether political consensus wishes to find individuals and the ideas they represent responsible for illegal or bad/destructive behavior. For example, for the Ft. Hood killer, a psychiatrist named Maj. Nidal M. Hasan, depictions were rife throughout major media claiming he was a sociopath or deranged, disturbed or unbalanced (or had social anxiety disorder or such, if they want to cite a DSM-5 disorder by name). Claiming murderers are "sociopaths" is to cite as cause an alleged mental disorder wherein a person lacks remorse or shame, who ignores the mores of his society and/or who was motivated by stress, per a typical headline in *The Washington Post* (November 7, 2009: "Psychiatric Stress Stretches Soldiers, System"). All such discussions vaguely or more precisely attribute such actions to mental causes over which the perpetrator has no control. There was no evidence in fact that the murders were motivated by anything other than agency: the choice to hate America, hate the military, and hate those he viewed as anti-Muslim. So he murdered over a dozen people and wounded an additional two dozen-plus.

In July of 2016, an African American ex-soldier murdered four police officers and a transit officer while wounding a dozen more, and, in negotiations related by Dallas Police Chief David Brown, the assassin, Micah Johnson, said he was "upset about the recent police shootings. The suspect said he was upset at white people. The suspect stated he wanted to kill white people, especially white officers" (Fernandez et al., 2016).

Yet, President Barack Obama insisted that the murderer was "demented," (Dennis et al., 2016) and the rhetoric of (invalidatable) mental illness explained the actions of the mass murderer Johnson for all those who had on their agenda the need to say his actions were not the result of human agency.

On CNN (July 11, 2016) Ron Hosko, FBI senior official, said that police were dialing back their aggressiveness, particularly if they are dealing with the "mentally ill." He said this plaintively, as if it were indisputable commonsense.

After the truck mass murder atrocity, claimed by ISIS as support for their terror aims, in Nice, France, "60 Minutes" did a piece introduced by Lesley

Stahl (July 17, 2016) in which she reported without editorial comment that the truck driver who intentionally plowed into "thousands of people" was said by his father to have "a history of mental illness." More conservative sources also speculated without comment on the possible/likely causality of mental problems in current terrorism. Such a perspective is omnipresent in media analysis from all political views when completely horrific but rational actions from the perpetrators' point of view are committed.

The fact is that virtually all national discussions of miscreant-caused mass murders and attempted mass murders include speculations that the accused was "mentally ill" or one of its synonyms ("troubled," "psychotic," "unbalanced," etc.). There is often debate as to whether said individuals are indeed mentally ill, but it is difficult and often impossible to find any public discussion or even consideration as to whether "mental illness" exists or is a myth.

Presidential candidate Donald Trump, representative of many people's typical reactions, said on the television news show *Meet the Press* and elsewhere regarding the shootings, "You have people who are mentally ill . . . they're going to do things that people believe are not even possible . . . [elsewhere] he said: "This isn't guns, this is about mental illness . . . [Y]ou have sick people in this country and throughout the world, and you're always going to have difficulty."

No one on the show countered this explanation. Ben Carson has blamed "mental disturbances"; Mike Huckabee has blamed mass killings on those who are "mentally deranged . . . do we need to do a better job on mental health? You bet we do" (NBC *Meet the Press*, October 4, 2015).

President Obama has blamed gun violence on "mental illnesses"; and former Senator Hillary Clinton, a strong supporter of parity coverage for mental illness and addiction treatment, is at the forefront of the argument that we need to pour more money into mental health care to stop violence in America, now that Tipper Gore is no longer the wife of a vice president. In other words, if there is anything on which the two major polarized parties are united, it is that mental illness exists, causes gun and other violence, must be combatted with more funding and seriousness and that therapy, defined as talk or drugs or both, must be available or required for those who have psychiatric illness. This is political science masquerading as medical science.

No presidential candidate to the knowledge of this writer has ever cast doubt on the existence of mental illness.

My own university classes, in which I teach the theories of mental illness, are perhaps prototypical of the public reactions. I have about

150 students in my "Persuasion" class at Towson University each year, white, black, rich, poor, middle-class, and every term, when I bring up Szasz, none of the students has ever heard of him. As I explain his view of the myth of mental illness, to be sure, many students find his way of thinking about behavior to be interesting and exciting, but invariably I get asked a variation on this question: "But what about people who really *are* mentally ill?"

With this question, they are generally asking about crazy behavior. Szasz has no problem with that: I personally asked him about forty years ago, "Tom, I know you don't believe in mental illness, but you do believe there are people who are just crazy, don't you?"

His answer: "And *how!*"

People cannot be convinced that there is no behavior that is unexplainable. They will not be convinced that they or their relatives are to blame for their misbehavior or inexplicable behavior. They will not be convinced in large numbers that professional psychological help for minors is not reasonable; can you leave parents with no options other than clergy, teachers, and friends? No, in untenable cases people have to believe that there are professionals who can work with malleable children's behaviors. That does not require the rhetorical armament of mental illness, but it does require counseling by any other name, and no significant number appears to want to rid the public of mental health counseling as an option. I myself believe that psychologists are often necessary to help wayward youth, although none of my children has ever gone that route.

Norman J. Ornstein, centrist writer for the American Enterprise Institute, wrote a piece for *The New York Times* near the end of 2015 called "How to Help Save the Mentally Ill from Themselves," (Ornstein, 2015). The op-ed article described the apoplexy a man has when his beloved son killed himself, perhaps accidentally, due to the lack of judgment of someone suffering from a mental illness who does not receive sufficient treatment, says Ornstein. There are no words that would convince a loving parent that his deceased son or daughter did not suffer from psychiatric illness or something that could have been cured or fixed by professional counseling.

Where the Myth of Mental Illness Is Believable

Are there any venues wherein the argument that mental illness is a myth is generally believable? Yes, wherein actors are motivated to believe in evil, the god-term of agency, such as the use of the insanity plea.

People who lose loved ones to violence or people who are distanced from perpetrators of violence are quite convincible regarding the outrage of the exculpation of criminals via insanity or "not criminally responsible" pleas.

Mafia boss Vincent Gigante's mental illness ruse in the latter 1900s which fooled a crew of Ivy League and other top psychologists and psychiatrists, did not convince prosecutor Charlie Rose, and almost everyone was surprised when he, Gigante, pursuant to a plea deal, admitted that he had faked his insanity (Vatz, 2003).

Moreover, only a few people believed that John Hinckley, a frequent target of Szasz's writing, was insane, and because of his unjust acquittal on the insanity plea, the presumption of such a plea, when allowed by the judge, was eliminated from federal trials.

Criminals throughout the United States have often been remanded to psychiatric care rather than tried for their criminal behavior, such as making threats. Often, the criminal justice system is abjured, as in the case of Andrew Goldstein, who, after committing over a dozen assaults on health care workers and other women, was always dealt with by the mental health system and never the criminal justice system. He had pushed a stranger, Kendra Webdale, off a platform into an oncoming train to her death. He stayed at the scene of the killing after his murderous action and waited, he said, to be sent for psychiatric care. Kendra's Law, enacted after the killing, forced some people into psychiatric treatment, but there was no movement before the atrocity to take criminal action against Goldstein. Perhaps if he had anticipated prison, he might have thought twice before committing the outrageous atrocity.

The lack of any widespread incredulity regarding drug usage as a mental illness is similar. *60 Minutes*, America's most sophisticated investigative television journalism, did a segment in December of 2015, on Michael Botticelli, the "drug czar," or the Director of National Drug Control Policy. The coverage was laudatory and cited the fact that he was a "recovering alcoholic." His philosophy, heralded widely, was a reiteration of all of the major responsibility-denying commonplaces that serve the myth of mental illness: said Botticelli, "Addiction is a brain disease. This is not a moral failing. This is not about bad people who are choosing to continue to use drugs because they lack willpower. You know, we don't expect people with cancer just to stop having cancer . . ." (*60 Minutes*, 2015).

Conclusion

Thomas Szasz's prolific writings and media work explicating why mental illness is a myth should be seen as an indisputable truth. Regardless, the responsibility-denying rhetoric of mental illness, steeped in mystification and self-serving explanations of the difficult-to explain, will perhaps forever successfully endure.

References

Blanco, C., Akudao, M., Wright, C., Hasin, D. S., Grand, B. F., Liu, S. –M. & Olfson, M. (December, 2008). Mental health of college students and their non-college-attending peers: Results from the National Epidemiologic Study on Alcohol and Related Conditions. *Archives of General Psychiatry,* 65, 1429–1437.

Dennis, B., & Wan, W. B. (July 9, 2016). Obama reaches out to battered nation after rage of 'demented' Dallas gunman. *The Washington Post.*

Fernandez, M., Pérez-Peña., R., & Bromwich, J. (July 8, 2016). Five dallas officers were killed as payback, police chief says. *The New York Times.* http://www.nytimes.com/2016/07/09/us/dallas-police-shooting.html?_r=0

"60 Minutes" (December 13, 2015). A new direction on drugs, http://www.cbsnews.com/news/60-minutes-a-new-direction-on-drugs/

Ornstein, N. J. (November 17, 2015). How to help save the mentally ill from themselves. *The New York Times.*

Stahl, L (July 17, 2016). "Bastille Day Tragedy," *"60 Minutes."* http://www.cbsnews.com/videos/bastille-day-tragedy/

Szasz, T. S. (1976). *Schizophrenia: The sacred symbol of psychiatry.* New York: Basic Books, Inc.

Szasz, T. S. (2010). *The myth of mental illness: Foundations of a theory of personal conduct.* New York: Harper Perennial.

Vatz, R. E. (May 20, 2003). Psychiatry in the courtroom. *The Washington Times.*

Vatz, R. E., & Weinberg, L. S. (1994). The rhetorical paradigm in psychiatric history: Thomas Szasz and the myth of mental illness. In M. S. Micale & R. Porter (Eds.), *Discovering the history of psychiatry.* Oxford: Oxford University Press.

Vatz, R. E., Weinberg, L. S., & Szasz, T. (September 15, 1985). Television and psychiatry? Outlook section of *The Washington Post.*

Part II

Exorcizing a Myth

4

Szasz's Distinction between Physical and Mental Illness

Joanna Moncrieff

Throughout his life and beyond Thomas Szasz was vilified for denying the suffering associated with what we currently refer to as "mental illness." "A legacy of denial of the seriousness of mental illness that has done more damage than good," was how one commentator put it in 2012, shortly after Szasz's death at the age of 92 (Warner, 2012). Others have accused him of denying the "reality" of mental illness and the distress it inevitably entails.

But Szasz never denied that the behaviors we refer to as "mental illness" could lead to anguish, misery, and harm. When writing about the "differences in behavior and speech" we call schizophrenia, for example, he highlighted how they could be "gravely disturbing to the so-called schizophrenic person, to those around him or to all concerned" (Szasz, 1988, p. 191).

Szasz's fundamental point is not that there are no real problems in need of addressing in some way, but that the particular range of problems we presently think of as "mental illness" are not rightly thought of as an illness. They are problems of a different kind from those that *are* correctly and appropriately called illnesses, and they require a different response. "In asserting that there is no such thing as mental illness I do not deny that people have problems coping with life and with each other," Szasz countered his critics in 1990 (Szasz, 1990, p. 135).

The fact that Szasz has been misread as suggesting that there are no problems to be dealt with, suggests how deeply ingrained the idea of mental illness is in modern society. We find it so difficult to conceptualize these problems in any other terms that we immediately interpret someone who says they are misconstrued as denying their very existence.

Szasz explained this situation too, through his recognition that the misrepresentation of the problems we refer to as mental illness as "illness" is strategic. In other words, it serves social and political purposes. The connotations of terms such as illness and disease, particularly the consensus that they are unwanted states of affairs determined by objective scientific enquiry, enables society to neutralize or manage problems that are designated as illness with little controversy or resistance. Labeling a challenging situation as an illness facilitates a certain sort of social response to the situation and to the individual who is identified as being the source of the problem.

Szasz argues that there is a fundamental distinction between the situations we refer to as physical disease, and those we call "mental illness." In his view the proper and coherent use of concepts such as "disease" and "illness" refer to conditions of the physical body. He pays little attention to what sort of bodily conditions might be referred to as diseases, and in what circumstances, because that is not his main interest. He takes the notion of physical disease as largely self-evident and uncontroversial, consisting of a deviation from the "structural and functional integrity of the human body" (Szasz, 1989, p. 12). At times he supported this notion by reference to the ideas of Rudolf Virchow, the nineteenth century pathologist (e.g., 2004, p. 51), who elaborated cell theory, and demonstrated that diseases could be characterized at the level of bodily structures like cells. For Virchow, a disease was an abnormality of a group, or multiple groups, of cells.

This simple concept of disease is not universally accepted however, and surveys show that there is considerable disagreement over what conditions qualify as diseases among and between medical professionals and lay people (Tikkinen et al., 2012; Campbell et al., 1979). The World Health Organization, which produces the International Classification of Disease, regards the terms "illness" and "disease" as so problematic that it does not even attempt to provide definitions (World Health Organisation, 1992). Problems with defining disease include how to classify common bodily conditions that do not necessarily cause direct physical suffering or shorten life (infertility, hypertension), as well as the issue of how to accommodate mental conditions. Recent debates about the nature of disease therefore center more on its outcomes than on the meaning of the concept itself.

The Social Consequences of the Disease Concept

Although official literature like the ICD shies away from the issue, Szasz correctly identified that the social arrangements that have developed for the care of people designated as sick or diseased arise from an underlying assumption that illness and disease are essentially conditions of the body.

Our responses to people who are sick arise from our understanding that bodily processes, as part of nature, are biologically programmed in ways over which we have no control, or at least little control. Biological processes follow their own predestined pathways, and are, most people believe, unamenable to human agency. Just as we are subject to the inexorable logic of biological aging, we cannot rid ourselves of cancer just because we wish to (or so most people believe, and science indicates). We cannot modify arthritis by strength of will.

This is not to deny that our mental state affects our body and vice versa. Emotions are expressed and experienced in the body as well as the mind. Acute anxiety may trigger a bodily event like fainting, a fit of anger may bring about a heart attack. Conversely, we may be able to modify the expression of certain physical states through acting on our body. We may be able to reduce pain or wheezing by exerting ourselves to relax, for example. We can also modify the expression of certain diseases through lifestyle changes, like giving up smoking, or eating a different diet and through physical or chemical intervention. We achieve these effects, however, by acting on our bodies, not through our choices or acts of will alone. None of this therefore contradicts the general understanding that bodily disease unfold according to its own biological principles, not to any human design or purpose.

The characteristics of the "sick role," described by Talcott Parsons, derive from the nature of diseases as autonomous biological processes. People who have diseases have privileges and exemptions from normal social expectations because of the recognition that biological events are not under human control (Parsons, 1951). The sick person is not held responsible for his or her condition or its consequences. Being sick is a morally neutral state, as opposed to behaving badly or inconsiderately. It is on this basis that the sick are considered worthy of care and attention. However, the sick person has to fulfill certain obligations in order to qualify for these entitlements. They have to accept their condition is undesirable, and they have to cooperate with a "competent treatment agent" (usually a doctor) (Conrad & Schneider, 1992, p. 32).

The extension of the "sick role" to include various forms of deviant behavior fulfills an important function in modern society. Designating an individual as sick justifies the allocation of public funds for care and subsistence through welfare payments like sickness and disability benefits, for example. The obligation on the sick person to get better also facilitates the management of forms of socially disruptive, dangerous or unwanted behavior that the criminal justice system finds difficult to manage. Since the sick person is not deemed to be criminally responsible, they are not meant to be punished, but their behavior can be changed by psychiatric intervention such as incarceration or the use of powerful, mind-altering drugs. In this way the psychiatric system can be seen as supplementing the formal criminal justice system and replacing the local, informal mechanisms for maintaining social order that existed for most of recorded history (Dershowitz, 1974). The "medicalization" of deviance also provides a mechanism for managing other social problems including childhood behavior problems, learning difficulties, addiction, and child abuse (Conrad & Schneider, 1992).

For many, the medicalization of problem behaviors represents a progressive, humanitarian response because it removes the moral approbation that would be attached to the behavior if it was regarded as willful. Whatever its advantages and disadvantages, however, many fundamental aspects of Western society depend on the designation of certain behavioral problems as illnesses. There are no accepted alternative mechanisms for supporting people who have difficulty coping with everyday life, or for managing many troublesome, but not obviously criminal behaviors.

If it turns out that what we regard as sickness is not necessarily located in the body, however, then the premises on which current societal procedures depend collapse. We are left with no established way of managing many taxing, but not extraordinary, social and interpersonal problems. What a disease is rightfully thought to be, and whether the concept should, or should not, include the problems we refer to as "mental illness," has hugely significant consequences.

Szasz on the Concepts of Disease and Illness

The heart of Szasz's critique of the concept of "mental illness" is the claim that "illness" and "disease" are terms whose core meaning derives from the body. The meaning of the two terms is closely related, but broadly we can say that "illness" refers to the experiences that arise in an individual as a result of a disease. Since illness derives from disease in this sense, I will concentrate on the concept of disease.

Surprisingly, the issue of whether or not a disease is necessarily a bodily condition has not been examined closely. This seems to be because it is either assumed to be the case, and discussion centers on how we view bodily processes, or because the issue is ignored.

The French philosopher of biology, Georges Canguilhem, states, for example, that "One can speak with reason of 'Greek Medicine' only from the Hippocratic period onward-that is to say from the moment when diseases came to be treated as bodily disorders" (Canguilhem, 2012). Others, however, simply assume that psychical, that is biological or bodily mechanisms, and "psychological mechanisms," that is thoughts and feelings, can be thought of as equivalent. Often the difficulties in distinguishing whether certain bodily states (like baldness or impotence) should qualify as diseases are conflated with the problem of conceptualizing nonbodily states as diseases. Psychiatrist Robert Kendall argues, for example, that "the differences between mental and physical illnesses, striking though some of them are, are quantitative rather than qualitative, differences of emphasis rather than fundamental differences" (Kendall, 2004, p. 42).

For Szasz, the term "disease," in its proper and coherent use, refers to changes in bodily structures or mechanisms that produce unwanted physical sensations and experiences, otherwise known as "symptoms." On this view, a disease, in its core sense, is an entity or process that is located in the physical body of the individual affected. In other words, a disease is a property of the biological system known as the body. "Illness," on this account, is the subjective experience that arises as a consequence of the presence of disease in the body.

In contrast, the situations referred to as "mental illness" consist of "patterns of personal conduct, unwanted by self or others" (Szasz, 2000). "Conduct" includes speech, which may reflect unusual or ungrounded beliefs, as well as dysfunctional or troublesome patterns of social interaction and functioning. The behavior may bother, threaten, or burden other people, as well as the individual affected.

It is human beings who think, speak, and act, not human bodies or brains. The problems designated as mental illness are consequently properties of human beings, not biological systems. Moreover, human behavior is only understandable in the context of the human society in which it is embedded. Behaviors regarded as characteristic of mental illness are deemed to be abnormal or problematic according to the particular circumstances in which they occur, and the norms of the society or group making the judgment. It may be acceptable, and indeed desirable, to show anger and aggression on the battlefield or in the boxing arena for example, but not toward strangers in the street. Similarly, a short attention span only becomes a problem with the introduction of a school system that demands sustained levels of attention from children at a young age. There is nothing intrinsically abnormal about the behaviors associated with mental illness. It is the circumstances in which they occur, and the social consequences they have, that define them as undesirable and problematic. Defining behavior as a "mental illness" is therefore to indicate the presence of a problem within a social system. For this reason Szasz referred to them as "problems in living" (Szasz, 1989, p. 12).

To illustrate the distinction, Szasz pointed out that most bodily diseases are also present in the dead body of the affected person: "almost every bodily illness a person can have, a cadaver can have too" (Szasz, 1990, p. 112). On the other hand, it makes no sense to assert that a cadaver has a mental illness. Szasz also repeatedly reminds us that once a bodily state or mechanism is identified that reliably distinguishes some people currently labeled as mentally ill from other people, the condition stops being regarded as a mental illness, and becomes a neurological "disease" instead. This, of course, assumes the pathology is located in the brain or nervous system; if the pathology was found to consist of a hormonal abnormality, for example, the condition would become an endocrinological disease. The principle remains the same, however— once a specific biological mechanism is identified, the condition is no longer conceived of as a mental illness. It is understood in terms of an abnormality, or disease, of the bodily system in which it is located.

Most symptoms of bodily disease are experienced in and by the body, or a part of the body; pain, breathlessness, and weakness, for example. The brain is a bodily organ too, however, and brain functioning is influenced by the condition of the rest of the body. Therefore, many common bodily diseases affect the way we think, including the common cold and a bout of "flu," both of which can impair our concentration and mental capacity.

Some diseases of the body affect people's thinking and behavior more profoundly, however, especially if they are located in the brain itself. There are usually, but not always, accompanying bodily manifestations. Thus, dementia produces a slow decline in cognitive abilities often accompanied by changes in behavior and mood. Physical symptoms such as slowness and weakness may be present, but may not be obvious. Multiple sclerosis and neurosyphilis can produce a distinctive change in personality, usually, and always eventually, accompanied by cognitive impairment and changes in mobility and balance.

Szasz recognized that behaviors may occasionally result from a putative neurological disease. He referred to syphilis and delirious states (e.g., drug intoxication) as conditions "in which persons may manifest certain disorders of thinking and behavior" (Szasz, 1989, p. 12). The fact that brain disease may affect behavior appears to present a problem for Szasz, however, since he wishes to draw a distinction between behavior (or conduct) and disease. If behavior *can* be a manifestation of disease, what is to counter the claim that *all* behaviors commonly classified as mental illness represent a disease?

Arguably, Szasz did not pay enough attention to the difficulties of pin-pointing the physical pathology underlying some diseases, and the occasional overlap between the symptoms of brain diseases or abnormalities, and those of mental disorders. Paying attention to how we identify "disease" in these marginal situations helps to clarify the distinctive features of the term, which guide its application, and the consequences that flow from it. It is not enough to simply describe the myriad ways in which the concepts of "disease" and "illness" are used in everyday language, however. Modern usage reflects many social and professional interests that have influenced the ways in which these concepts are applied. We need instead to pay attention to the distinctions that people make, and the consequences that flow from these distinctions.

Disease at the Margins

The bodily processes that produce what we regard as brain diseases are not always identifiable. The pathology underlying multiple sclerosis, for example, has only become visible since the advent of Magnetic Resonance Imaging (MRI). The brain changes that produce what we call "dementia" are not qualitatively different from the changes that occur in normal aging; they are simply more exaggerated. You cannot distinguish the brain of an individual with Alzheimer's disease or vascular dementia from one without, even though, as a group, people with dementia have more brain pathology.

Yet we accepted that multiple sclerosis is a brain disease long before MRI came along. There must, therefore, be other criteria on which we base our judgments about whether or not something qualifies as a bodily disease. Similarly, the diagnosis of dementia remains one that is based on observable signs and symptoms. Yet, there has never been any controversy about whether multiple sclerosis or dementia constitutes brain disorders. They are regarded as just as much bodily conditions as heart disease or lung cancer. We assume, for example, that they remain present in the body of the affected individual after death. Our confidence about the status of dementia and multiple sclerosis as brain diseases therefore suggests there are clinical features that lead us to assume the presence of an underlying brain process, which are independent of whether or not this process can be visualized or detected in the human brain.

Epilepsy is another useful example. In between fits, the brains of many people with epilepsy are normal (as revealed by an electroencephalogram (EEG), MRI, or any other technique for revealing brain structure or function). If you do an EEG during a fit, it is usually abnormal, but it simply isn't possible for everyone with epilepsy to be wired up to an EEG machine until they have a fit. Even then, some people do not show any abnormalities, because the EEG doesn't detect signals over the relevant area, or the activity causing the fit is buried too deep in the brain.

Like multiple sclerosis or dementia, we have little problem in deciding that epilepsy is a disease. If, however, we think that an individual is intentionally initiating behavior that looks like epileptic fits, we do not regard this as epilepsy. In fact, we have a separate name for this situation; we call it "pseudo-epilepsy." It appears to be the case, therefore that in "real" epilepsy, we assume that the abnormal experiences (fits) arise from disordered brain activity. When people have pseudo-epileptic seizures, we think they are deliberately or purposively imitating epilepsy.

Similarly, people may develop paralysis of their limbs in a variety of bodily diseases, and the underlying pathology may not be identifiable in every case. However, sometimes people deliberately imitate paralysis, for their own conscious or subconscious purposes. This situation is sometimes referred to as "hysteria," (now officially named "conversion disorder"), Munchausen's disease (now called "factitious disorder") or malingering, depending on the level to which conscious as opposed to unconscious motivation is believed to be involved. Where the paralysis is believed to be the result of a brain lesion, it is understood to have arisen from a spontaneous bodily process that occurs independently of the individual's agency or will. In the case of hysteria or malingering, the sufferer is believed to have initiated the paralysis of his own accord. The hysteric could walk if he decided to, at least there is no bodily lesion or process that prevents him from doing so.

Although it may not always be possible to make the distinction, it is clear that we regard paralysis that is due to a stroke as different from hysterical paralysis or malingering. These situations require different interventions or treatments and suggest the need for differing social and interpersonal responses. We might, for example, discourage the provision of appliances, such as wheelchairs, to people with hysteria or Munchausen's disease for fear of prolonging their symptoms and increasing dependency. We would certainly not want to treat a person with pseudoepileptic seizures with antiepileptic medication.

Detecting Disease

The effort we put into identifying whether a condition originates in the body or not provides further evidence that physical illness and mental illness denote different sorts of situations and that the distinction is important.

If we are trying to work out whether a person having "fits" has an epileptic brain disease, or whether they are deliberately mimicking epilepsy, we immediately look for recognized physical signs. These are observable bodily reactions or states that are not present, or not usually present, in healthy people, and have been established to be associated with the disease in question. In other words, we look for evidence that the origin of the disorder is the body. So if someone bites his tongue and urinates during a fit, we would be more confident that it is a genuine epileptic fit than if he does not. If someone with paralysis shows the Babinski sign (a reflex, when the toes of the foot curl up instead of down), we would suspect it is due to brain pathology, rather than being a hysterical state.

Some mental states are also accepted as being indicative of a bodily condition. Cognitive decline or "dementia" is so closely associated with conditions affecting the brain that we practically view this state as a physical sign. If someone is born with limited cognitive abilities, we also view this as arising from a deficiency in brain functioning, whether or not a specific defect can be identified. In most cases of intellectual disability, incidentally, it cannot.

There are similar lessons if we look at situations where brain diseases mimic mental disorders; that is situations involving "symptoms" we normally associate with mental disorder, like mood changes or behavioral disturbance, which transpire to arise from a brain condition. In the early stages of dementia, for example, people can develop paranoid ideas and depression that are indistinguishable from other cases of psychosis or depression in older people. Occasionally, bizarre behavior and psychotic symptoms will be the outstanding feature in people with an acute brain condition like encephalitis. In both of these cases we look for signs of a bodily origin to the disorder in order to decide on the nature of the problem. As Szasz pointed out, when and if we can attribute the behavior to a physical condition, we rule out understanding the situation as what we usually understand by a mental illness or disorder. We also rule out ordinary, purposive, voluntary action, that is the conscious production of physical symptoms to achieve some goal or personal gain, which may be referred to as "malingering."

The other way we attempt to discriminate between situations that arise from a brain disease and those that do not is by asking whether the behavior is understandable. If we can fathom a motive for the behavior, or understand it as a meaningful response to external events, then we would be less inclined to view it as arising from a bodily disease. Hence we may come to suspect that the person with pseudo-seizures has learnt that having fits is associated with positive attention, care, and getting off school or work, for example. Drug addicts sometimes fake epileptic fits in order to obtain the sedative drugs that are used to treat them. If an elderly person has just undergone a life-changing event such as the death of a spouse, or retirement, then we would be more inclined to believe they were in a depressed state than demonstrating the early signs of dementia.

Although we want to distinguish these situations, tests on the body, such as blood tests and brain imaging, may not be definitive. Investigations may appear to be normal in people who later transpire to have a bodily condition, and may show nonspecific abnormalities in people who most likely have hysteria or depression or some other mental disorder diagnosis.

Although it may not always be possible to come to a definitive conclusion, it is clear that conceptually we find it important to make a distinction between cases in which there is, or is likely to be, a bodily condition that explains behaviors or "symptoms," and cases where there is not. Looking at situations in which this distinction is challenging only confirms that we go to some lengths to distinguish between behavior that is driven by internal biological processes (diseases) that are independent of the individual's will, and behavior that is initiated by the individual themselves. Making this distinction matters.

"Mental Symptoms"

As mentioned earlier, cognitive dysfunction or intellectual impairment is universally regarded as a symptom of brain disease. It is useful to look further at the differences between cognitive dysfunction and other "mental symptoms" to elucidate when and why a certain pattern of thinking or behavior is incontrovertibly associated with brain dysfunction. No one has suggested, to my knowledge, that cognitive decline might be an understandable reaction to life events, or a complex but meaningful response to perceived threats or difficulties, for example. The fact that cognitive impairment, in later life at least, is progressive may account for some of our intuition that it arises from a brain disorder, but the intellectual impairment that occurs from birth is usually static. Yet we have the same inclination that intellectual disability originates in the brain.

Even before we could confirm that cognitive impairment is associated with various types of brain pathology, it seems to have been understood differently from other mental symptoms, on the basis of its particular character. Thus in 1938, for example, Jaspers distinguished the cognitive abnormalities found in the condition known as General Paralysis or General Paralysis of the Insane (a neurological condition caused by syphilis, characterized by dementia and behavioral abnormalities) with the symptoms of "schizophrenia" as follows: "in the one case it is as if an axe had destroyed a piece of clockwork, and crude destructions are of little interest. In the other it is as if the clockwork keeps going wrong, stops and then runs again." This appears to suggest simply that schizophrenia involves a more superficial and temporary brain dysfunction, and he went on to say: "but there is more than that. The schizophrenic life is peculiarly productive. In certain cases, the very manner of it, its contents and all that it represents can in itself create another kind of interest. We find ourselves astounded and shaken in the presence of alien secrets, which in this sense cannot possibly happen when we are faced with the crude destructions, irritations and excitements of General Paralysis" (Jaspers, 1968, p. 576) cited in (Jenner et al., 1993, p. 32).

Thus although Jaspers believed that the somatic basis of conditions like schizophrenia would one day be revealed, he also suggested that "Even when we have discovered the somatic processes underlying the psychoses, there will always persist a profound contrast between the various different psychoses [in which class he included General Paralysis], and probably too an interest of quite a different order in their psychic aspects" (Jaspers, 1968, p. 576) cited in (Jenner et al., 1993, p. 32).

Therefore it seems that it is not just the empirical association with specific brain pathologies that suggests to us that cognitive impairment is indicative of a biological condition, nor its progressive course when it occurs in later life. It seems to be something about its depleting nature: something about the fact that there is loss or lack without gain;

a narrowing and restriction of human capacities, a lowering of the qualities that we associate with full human mental functioning, with no compensation in terms of the creation of alternative ways of seeing or responding to the world.

In contrast, the individual in the grip of a paranoid psychosis can be extraordinarily creative in constructing a delusional system or interpreting their own thoughts as alien occurrences. Even the fragmented and elusive speech of people with thought disorder can be made to make some sense, usually of a tangential kind that suggests a creative process of sorts. And depression too, despite the reduced functioning that it often entails, involves a productive state of self-blaming, catastrophizing, and pessimistic interpretations of the world. This is not meant to suggest that psychosis or depression are productive or useful states as we usually understand the term "productive." The idea that mental disorders represent a privileged view on the world has been criticized for over-romanticizing mental disorders, with some merit, although I would also agree with the view that there may sometimes be insights to be gained from unusual and extreme experiences. Here I am simply making the point that states of madness or emotional extremis are not simply states of deficiency, as the state of cognitive decline or impairment can be understood to be. Unlike someone with dementia, people with psychosis or severe depression have not lost the tools of mental activity. They are merely employing those tools in unusual ways.

It seems to be the loss or "lack" indicated by a state such as dementia that, unlike other mental symptoms, signals the likely presence of an underlying brain condition. Sometimes severe mental illness can mimic this state, as with negative symptoms of schizophrenia or a depressive stupor. In such circumstances, however, mental abilities remain intact, and inklings of productive and creative thought can be witnessed in periods of remission or in response to particular stimuli. I recall a young man with severe negative state schizophrenia, for example, who barely spoke, and spent almost all of his time slumped in a chair with his hood drawn down, apparently doing nothing. He could, however, rouse himself to levels of extraordinary ingenuity in order to obtain supplies of marijuana!

Responses to the Myth of Mental Illness

For a long time now it has been fashionable to dismiss Szasz's differentiation between physical disease and "mental illness" as outdated and superseded. It is often derided as "dualist" with vague intonations about the interaction of mind and body.

There are two broad theoretical positions from which such criticisms arise. In the first, it is claimed that mental disorders are in fact brain diseases, just like multiple sclerosis, but ones in which the underlying pathology has not yet been identified. In the second, the concept of disease is redefined, dislocating it from its association with the physical body, and relating it instead to vague concepts like dysfunction, or adaptation.

Mental Illness as Putative Brain Disease

As Szasz points out, the notion of "mental illness" ultimately derives its legitimacy from the idea that the disorders it refers to *might* originate from a brain disease (Szasz, 1989). The fact that there are occasional cases like syphilis, or encephalitis, as referred to before, in which a neurological condition turns out to be present in people with the sort of abnormal behaviors that are usually classified as a "mental illness" is frequently cited to support this case. It is also regularly claimed, although with little foundation, that the physical basis of mental conditions like schizophrenia has already been identified.

This claim is not true. Differences between the brains of people diagnosed with a mental disorder and so-called "healthy controls" occur for a variety of reasons and do not necessarily indicate that the source of the condition has been identified. The mentally ill subjects in brain studies are usually recruited from hospital populations, which include the most disturbed and impaired individuals. The healthy controls are often members of hospital staff. Patients' intelligence quotient (IQ) is usually lower than the control group, and IQ is associated with brain size (Deary et al., 2010); patients are taking medication, which changes the brain, and patients in institutions have less stimulating environments than other people, which may also affect brain structure. In any case, none of the differences so far identified are specific. They are present in many people without a diagnosed mental illness, and are found across different types of mental disorder.

In fact, the most consistently demonstrated abnormalities in the brains of people with a particular mental disorder, the smaller brain size and larger brain cavities of people diagnosed with schizophrenia compared with controls, are at least partially, and maybe totally, attributable to the effects of antipsychotic medication (Moncrieff & Leo, 2010). Any residual differences are likely due to differences in IQ, which has rarely been adequately controlled.

As Szasz pointed out, it may transpire that some forms of what is currently diagnosed as mental illness are ultimately detected to have a specific underlying pathology. In this case, they would legitimately be regarded as brain diseases. Highly sensitive and sophisticated methods of exploring the brain have so far failed to reveal any specific abnormalities associated with conditions like schizophrenia or depression, however. Indeed, nothing resembling a specific biological marker of any "mental illness" has ever been found, even in the era of such penetrating technology such as MRI.

There is another more philosophical problem with this position however. Although we can accept that there are occasional cases in which behavior originates in a brain abnormality, it is highly problematic to suggest that all the behaviors that fall under the rubric of mental illness are driven by impersonal biological mechanisms in this way. Do all the people currently diagnosed as depressed and started on antidepressants really feel their feelings and behavior are under the alien control of their serotonin or noradrenaline levels, or the structure of their brain's hippocampus? And since there is no categorical division between the feelings that can be diagnosed as "major depressive disorder" and ordinary depression or sadness, does this not imply that all feelings and thoughts are beyond our control, that human existence is merely the playing out of a preset biological program? As critics of this sort of reductionist determinism have pointed out, the idea that human beings are free, self-determining agents is so deeply embedded in our understanding of the world that denying it renders our language and activity meaningless and incomprehensible (Berlin, 1954).

Redefining Disease

The other response to Szasz's position is to redraw the boundaries of disease. This has been attempted in the context of a debate about whether "disease" is an objective, empirical concept that simply exists in the world, or whether it is a normative or evaluative concept that is dependent on human judgment.

Peter Sedgwick, among other thinkers, points out that there are no diseases in nature (Sedgwick, 1982). Just as weeds are defined by gardeners, diseases are situations that are defined as unwanted from the point of view of the sufferer and depend on his or her particular social context. Malaria is bad for humans, but good for the malaria parasite, for example. Moreover, chronic malaria is so common in parts of Africa it is regarded as normal. It is only when higher levels of productivity and more regular, Western style working patterns are demanded, that it starts to become a problem.

74

The pharmaceutical industry can manipulate human perceptions to create diseases where there were previously none. Hence normal, often age-related variation in sexual functioning can be presented as a disease—that is as something that is undesirable and needs to be corrected.

Whether the body functions adequately depends on its environment and the demands it has to meet, and these depend on the particular conventions and expectations of a given society. Those authors that stress the evaluative nature of disease are right to identify that simply being a feature of the body is not *enough* to qualify something as a disease. There is also a value judgment involved about the consequences of that condition and the benefits of treating it, which will differ from one context to another. But these writers take the argument a step further and suggest that it is the disvalued nature of disease that is central to the concept, and therefore that other situations involving a negative value judgment can also be called a disease. This is tantamount to saying that any unwanted situation can be considered to be a disease.

Philosopher and psychiatrist Bill Fulford's definition of illness, for example, is that of "action failure" (Fulford, 1989). This, he explains, is a failure of fully developed "ordinary doing," by which he means the way human beings act in accordance with goals and purposes, although usually not in an explicitly conscious manner. We behave in ways that are consistent with our aims and interests, for example, but most of the time we do this unconsciously. It is only when confronted by conflicting possibilities that we have to reflect or deliberate on our choices and actions.

For Fulford, physical and mental conditions qualify as "illnesses" because both restrict "ordinary doing." In the case of bodily conditions this restriction comes about through bodily weakness, pain, or other physical disabilities. In mental illness, according to Fulford, there is a failure of agency, so that people are also unable to act according to their aims and purposes as they usually would.

Fulford recognizes that agency is a key problem in mental disorders, and this allows him to elide mental and physical illness by suggesting that the term "illness" demarcates a situation in which an individual's agency is compromised. In his terms therefore, illness equates to "action failure."

Despite wanting to bring mental disorders and physical diseases together under the same concept of "illness," Fulford recognizes that they are different and distinctive situations. Moreover, he is right to pinpoint the essential relation between disease or illness and agency, and that the question of agency is a key problem in considering the nature of mental disorders. However, he overlooks the fact that the origins of the relation between disease and lack of moral agency derives from the nature of the body and the autonomy of our biological nature. The failure of agency caused by physical illness is quite different from the subtle and complex way that intention is molded and manifested in mental disorders (as discussed in more detail below). In the former situation, a person's conscious intention (to stand up or go to work) is straightforwardly thwarted by the weakness or dysfunctionality of the body (pain, dizziness, fatigue, etc.). In the latter, the individual's intentions are complex and conflicted, but the behavior is still an expression of the individual's purposive nature, even if it does not fulfill all his or her conscious motivations.

Wakefield's much-discussed concept of "harmful dysfunction" is another attempt to change the boundaries of disease to accommodate mental disorders (Wakefield, 1992). It also represents a response to authors like Sedgewick and Fulford, in trying to put the concepts of disease and illness back onto an objective empirical foundation. Wakefield elides bodily dysfunction and psychological dysfunction by presenting both as objective entities that can be defined by a failure to fulfill evolutionary purposes. The highly reductionist implication of Wakefield's idea, which is not spelt out explicitly, is that psychological functions are produced by evolutionarily adapted biological mechanisms *and* can therefore be equated to those biological mechanisms. As with the idea that human behavior is driven by brain chemicals or genes, we end up with a depleted view of the nature of human existence that renders nonsensical our everyday understanding of human beings as autonomous agents.

Wakefield's reliance on evolutionary theory has also been criticized in its application to biological disease mechanisms. Schaffner, for example, argues that medicine uses mechanistic not adaptive explanations of function. Thus we define normal cardiac function as the level of functioning required to keep the rest of the body alive and well, and there is no need to postulate natural selection or an evolutionary teleology (Schaffner, 1993). Moreover, evolutionary psychology is a highly questionable basis for objectivity. It has been shown to be shot through with evaluative judgments about what "normal," "natural," or "proper" mental functions, and their behavioral expressions, consist of (Houts, 2001).

Szasz did not deny, as is sometimes implied, that the concepts of disease and illness are normative. He merely observed that wanted or unwanted, bodily conditions can be described in empirical, objective terms: "although the desirability of physical health, as such, is an ethical norm, what health is can be stated in anatomical and physiological terms" (Szasz, 1989, p. 14). In contrast, attempts to extend notions of disease and illness beyond the body, as Fulford and Wakefield's positions illustrate, end up with concepts that simply refer to an undesirable state of affairs. In terms of formal logic, although being a condition of the body may be *insufficient* to mark something as a disease, it is surely, at least, *necessary*. For the term disease to be clear and useful, it must be able to distinguish a certain set of unwanted situations from others. Being a biological condition of the body is a minimum requirement for a coherent concept of what we call "disease." Divorced from the body, illness and disease can be applied to so many unwanted situations they cease to have any discriminative power. They become meaningless.

What Is Mental Illness? Inexplicability and the Problem of Agency

As illustrated earlier, it appears that we do want to distinguish between situations that are caused by a condition located in the body, and those produced by the self-initiated action of an individual. We normally discern that a behavior is a self-initiated action by determining the purpose or meaning of the action—what goal it is directed to achieving, for example, or what circumstance it is a response to.

The behavior that characterizes mental illness is challenging in this respect, however. It may be difficult to detect the purpose of the behavior, or to understand the relation between the behavior and its context. The behavior and utterances we refer to as "mental illness" may be, or appear to be, "inexplicable" or "irrational." In other words, they seem to lack an obvious purpose. Indeed, it seems that inexplicability is a characteristic feature of the behaviors and situations referred to as madness, lunacy, or insanity over the centuries. Today too, as sociologist Jeff Coulter explores, it is the incomprehensible nature of certain patterns of behavior that triggers lay ascriptions of mental illness, and it is these lay judgments that determine the deviant status of the situation rather than any technical, scientific procedures (Coulter, 1979).

Humans naturally seek explanations for events. When we cannot understand the motive for behavior—when someone does something "out of the blue" or for no apparent reason—we may be inclined to explain the situation by presuming that the behavior is the result of an autonomous biological process, operating in isolation from the ordinary will of the individual. This was the basis on which Jaspers declared that the "psychoses" were disorders of biological origin.

Psychosis is the name currently applied to various states in which people appear to have lost contact with reality. It is an umbrella term, which includes schizophrenia, alongside other psychotic states, such as drug-induced reactions. It is often characterized by hallucinations and delusions (unsubstantiated beliefs, which unlike religious beliefs, are not explicable in terms of culture). People often misinterpret events around them as being personally significant. Although rarely transparent, the meaning of psychotic states has been explored by sufferers and observers alike. The psychoanalytical explanation of paranoia as a projection of personal insecurities represents one such attempt, present in the writings of Freud and other early analysts (Bone & Oldham, 1994). This approach is endorsed by first-person accounts of paranoid delusions, which illustrates the way they can operate to counteract low self-esteem and expectations by boosting self-significance (May, 2001).

R. D. Laing explored the meaning of psychotic states in more general terms, seeing them as an expression of existential anxiety, and an attempt to protect the self from dissolution. On this account, the internal fantasy world of the psychotic provides an appealing alternative to the real world of conflicting and overwhelming demands (Laing, 1965). We also have an increasing volume of testimony by people who have suffered psychotic breakdowns on the meaning of their symptoms; many (though not all) relating them to past experiences of trauma or abuse (Hornstein, 2009).

Social constructivists have also revealed how emotions, or at least the behavior by which we express our emotions, have a communicative, and therefore purposive, function (Harre, 1986). Feeling sad about an event may be involuntary, but acting in a depressed fashion can be understood as a meaningful response to an unfortunate situation, and as a way of communicating our feelings to others and invoking a response from those around us.

As alluded to above, Fulford is right to identify that at the heart of the question about the nature of mental disorder is the question of agency, or intentionality. If an event, such as a "fit" or seizure occurs because of an underlying biological condition, like epilepsy, we do not regard it as intentional. Calling a condition an illness or disease implies that the individual affected has no control over its manifestations. The "symptoms" are not the result of purposive or intentional action. The intentionality of the individual who behaves in a way we characterize as mentally ill, however, is problematic. The behavior does not seem to be straightforwardly purposive and "motivated" in the sense that ordinary voluntary behavior is motivated. People do not choose to be depressed or psychotic like they might chose to take up a new hobby. The individual may be unaware of their motivations and unable to account for their actions, for example; they likely have conflicting motivations; they may have paid little attention to all the potential consequences of their behavior. They may have trouble controlling their level of emotional arousal, making considered decision-making more challenging. Yet it is possible to find meaning in madness, if we probe deeply enough into a person's life history and circumstances, and if we suspend our own normative judgments about sensible and appropriate ways to behave.

Fulford uses the example of "compulsive behavior," such as people show in drug or alcohol addiction or "obsessive compulsive disorder" (OCD), to illustrate the state that he calls "action failure." In this state he argues, people are unable to act in the ways they intend because they are thwarted by an inner compulsion (Fulford, 1989).

Fulford highlights the difficulty we have in attributing full agency to an individual who acts in a compulsive manner; the individual who continues to drink when he knows it will kill him, for example. But we all do things we know are not good for us now and again (in fact very often, if you are a fairly ordinary human being). We all act "impulsively" in some situations and then look back on it and regret that we did not consider the consequences of our choices more fully. We all have conflicting motives in many circumstances—wanting to have another drink because we like the effect, but not wanting to damage our health; wanting to help someone but wanting to satisfy our own needs too. Many people feel they lack the self-control they would like when it comes to eating, smoking or sex. Many suffer from anxiety in certain situations, which limits their activities to some extent. We all feel at some points that we lack the stamina to persist in tedious or demanding tasks that we know will be useful in the long run.

Moreover, little of our ordinary, everyday behavior involves the sort of considered reflection that we associate with fully rational decision-making and we often behave in ways that are inconsistent with our stated or conscious goals and purposes. Nevertheless, we still consider our everyday behavior to consist of our own, voluntarily initiated actions. In this sense then, the compulsive behavior that characterizes disorders like addictions is an extreme variant of a pattern of behavior we recognize and are familiar with. It is part and parcel of "ordinary doing" as Fulford calls it, and not its opposite or failure (Fulford, 1989).

Compulsive behavior with its mixed motivations is a good model for other sorts of mental disorders, I believe. It allows us to see meaning in the behaviors associated with mental disorders, but simultaneously to understand that these are not simple choices. It also enables us to encourage the individual to find their own resources with which to resist and counteract behaviors that have become problematic.

In depression, for example, the individual has conflicting motives. She knows she should get up and go to work, play with her children, or join her friends for a social occasion, but it feels like too much effort and she is afraid she will not be able to cope. On the one hand she knows she needs to sort out the credit card bills that made her depressed in the first place, on the other hand she does not want to because thinking about the problem makes her feel worse. Or she may not be able to work out why she is feeling low in the first place. She may have a nagging suspicion, but she is afraid to focus on it too much in case it is overwhelming.

Psychosis, too, is understandable in these terms. The attractions of psychosis are more difficult to fathom, but they are not nonexistent. Withdrawing into an internal fantasy life blocks out the challenges and anxieties provoked by the real world. Psychosis can be a vivid and colorful place, where the individual feels real and valued (even if they also feel persecuted), which can provide an escape from feelings of insignificance and inadequacy experienced in the real world.

From this perspective, the behaviors we refer to as mental disorders are meaningful; which is to say they serve some purpose. The purpose is often not easy to fathom, either for the individual or those around her. The purpose served by the "mentally ill" behavior also likely conflicts with the individual's other intents and purposes. We have difficulty conceptualizing agency in anything other than binary terms, however. The behaviors associated with mental disorders are not driven by impersonal biological mechanisms that unfold independently of the individual's intentions, but neither do they conform to some ideal of carefully considered intentional action.

We can recognize in our own, everyday "ordinary doing" that our motivations are often complex, conflicting, and opaque. Agency in mental disorder is complex and compromised in the same ways. Unwanted as they may often be, the "symptoms" of mental disorder are an intrinsic part of the individual self that manifests them. The bizarre, irrational and apparently incomprehensible states that we currently sweep under the umbrella of "mental illness," are a manifestation of the plethora of purposive human activity.

Admitting agency back into the situations we call "mental illness" immediately opens a Pandora's box of problems, however. Whereas we may be able to accept a situation in which a diseased person is incarcerated for their own good, the idea of forcibly changing the voluntary behavior of individuals outside the criminal justice system, is anathema to a modern, liberal democratic system. It also calls into question the basis for allocating public welfare, if the behavior at issue is acknowledged as belonging to the individual, and not attributable to external biological forces.

The Survival of the Mental Illness Concept

There are many reasons why individuals, groups, or society may want to designate certain problems as "illness." People may wish to explain their difficulties in living up to social expectations; people or society may want to control the unwanted behavior of others; people want and need care, and most modern societies, thankfully, do not like to see people destitute. All these things are facilitated by defining them as "illness," because an illness is regarded as a bodily process that is, by its biological nature, beyond the will of the individual to redress. The social significance of the concept of "illness" derives from its association with the body.

The social function of the idea of "mental illness" is the key to why it has endured for so long, and not any claim to scientific integrity. Finding alternative approaches to address the vast array of problems that now come under its umbrella, which are compatible with modern values of freedom and humanitarianism, is not easy. Szasz himself acknowledged that he did not know how else to manage the issue of "adult dependency," for example.[1] Yet, the first step to devising alternative strategies must be to acknowledge the nature of the problems involved. Adult dependency is one of them. How society should respond to seemingly incomprehensible (irrational), troublesome, and sometimes dangerous behavior is another. The "myth of mental illness" only conceals the nature and complexity of these problems, by presenting them as objective biological states located in individuals. By obscuring the manner in which these are problems of, and for, social groups and systems it prevents us from devising more transparent social processes that attempt to balance the interests of all parties affected by these testing "problems of living."

Note

1. Szasz made a comment to this effect during the International Network for Philosophy and Psychiatry held in Manchester in 2010.

References

Berlin, I. (1954). *Historical inevitability.* London: Oxford University Press.

Bone, S., & Oldham, J. S. (1994). *Paranoia: New psychoanalytic perspectives.* Madison, CT: International Universities Press.

Campbell, E. J., Scadding, J. G., & Roberts, R. S. (1979). The concept of disease. *British Medical Journal, 2,* 757–762.

Canguilhem, G. (2012). *Writings on medicine (forms of living).* New York: Fordham University Press.

Conrad, P., & Schneider, J. W. (1992). *Deviance and medicalization: From badness to sickness.* Philadelphia, PA: Temple University Press.

Coulter, J. (1979). *The social construction of mind.* London: Macmillan.

Deary, I. J., Penke, L., & Johnson, W. (2010). The neuroscience of human intelligence differences. *Nature Reviews Neuroscience, 11,* 201–211.

Dershowitz, A. (1974). The origins of preventive confinement in anglo-american law- Part 1: The English experience. *University of Cincinnati Law Review, 43,* 1–60.

Fulford, K. W. M. (1989). *Moral theory and medical practice.* Cambridge: Cambridge University Press.

Harre, R. (1986). An outline of the social constructionist viewpoint. In R. Harre (Ed.), *The social construction of emotions* (pp. 2–14). London: Blackwell

Hornstein, G. (2009). *Agnes's jacket: A psychologist's search for the meaning of madness.* New York: Rodale.

Houts, A. C. (2001). Harmful dysfunction and the search for value neutrality in the definition of mental disorder: Response to Wakefield, part 2. *Behaviour Research and Therapy, 39,* 1099–1132.

Jaspers, K. (1968). *General psychopathology* (J. Hoenig & M.W. Hamilton, Trans.) Manchester: Manchester University Press.

Jenner, F. A., Monteiro, A. C. D., Zagalo-Cardoso, J. A., & Cunha-Oliveira, J. A. (1993). *Schizophrenia: A disease or some ways of being human.* Sheffield: Sheffield Academic Press.

Kendall, R. E. (2004). The myth of mental illness. In J. A. Schaler (Ed.), *Szasz under fire* (pp. 29–48). Chicago: Open Court.

Laing, R. D. (1965). *The divided self.* London: Pelican Books.

May, R. (2001). Taking a stand: Fergus Keane interview with Rufus May. BBC radio 4, 6th February 2001 [On-line].

Moncrieff, J., & Leo, J. (2010). A systematic review of the effects of antipsychotic drugs on brain volume. *Psychological Medicine, 40,* 1409–1422.

Parsons, T. (1951). *The social system.* London: Routledge and Keegan Paul.

Schaffner, K. F. (1993). *Discovery and explanation in biology and medicine.* Chicago, IL: University of Chicago Press.

Sedgwick, P. (1982). *Psychopolitics*. London: Harper & Row.

Szasz, T. (1988). *Schizophrenia. The sacred symbol of psychiatry*. Syracuse, NY: Syracuse University Press.

Szasz, T. (1989). *Law, liberty and psychiatry: An inquiry into the social uses of mental health*. Syracuse, NY: Syracuse University Press.

Szasz, T. (1990). *The untamed tongue*. Chicago: Open Court.

Szasz, T. (2000). Mental disorders are not diseases. *USA Today*, January.

Szasz, T. (2004). Reply to Kendall. In J. A. Schaler (Ed.) (pp. 49–55). Chicago: Open Court.

Tikkinen, K. A., Leinonen, J. S., Guyatt, G. H., Ebrahim, S., & Jarvinen, T. L. (2012). What is a disease? Perspectives of the public, health professionals and legislators. *BMJ Open, 2*, e001632–e001632.

Wakefield, J. C. (1992). Disorder as harmful dysfunction: A conceptual critique of DSM-III-R's definition of mental disorder. *Psychological Review, 99*, 232–247.

Warner, J. (2012). The denial of mental illness is alive and well. [On-line]. Available: http://ideas.time.com/2012/09/14/the-denial-of-mental-illness-is-alive-and-well/

World Health Organisation (1992). *The ICD-10 classification of mental and behvioural disorders*. Geneva: World Health Organisation.

5

What Follows from the Nonexistence of Mental Illness?

David Ramsay Steele   p. ᒿ ᵊ ᒑ

Does Thomas Szasz's opposition to psychiatric coercion follow from his denial of the existence of mental illness? My question isn't whether either or both of these Szasz positions are correct, but whether one implies the other.

In 1961 Szasz published *The Myth of Mental Illness* (amplifying an article with the same title, from a year earlier). His subsequent books, nearly forty of them, would all preach the same message. Szasz maintained that there is literally no such thing as "mental illness." Illness is a condition of the body, and mental illness is no more than a metaphor (Szasz, 1991, p. 23, 2007, pp. 3–4, 2010, p. 267). "Because the mind is not a bodily organ, it can be diseased only in a metaphorical sense" (Szasz, 2001, p. 13).

Equally consistently, Szasz held that treating people against their will is unwarranted and immoral. He argued and actively campaigned against all coercion by the state in the name of mental health. He opposed involuntary commitment of the "mentally ill," all compulsory treatment of adults, and all legal restrictions on voluntary ingestion of chemical substances, from tobacco to crystal meth (Szasz, 2001, pp. 127–165).

Szasz evidently believed that there is a tight connection between the proposition that there is literally no such thing as mental illness and the proposition that all psychiatric coercion is wrong, or at least unjustified. Again and again he reveals that he assumes some such tight connection (1976, p. 189, 2010, pp. 267–268), but he never spells out an argument demonstrating this connection.

It might seem at first blush that, since the case for psychiatric coercion is usually made in terms of the reality of mental illness, to refute the existence of mental illness would automatically destroy the case for psychiatric coercion. But since proponents of psychiatric coercion generally view the reality of mental illness as uncontentious, they naturally talk in terms of mental illness. This doesn't demonstrate that the literal existence of mental illness is crucial to their support for coercion. We can imagine people convinced by Szasz's arguments that there is no literal mental illness continuing to hold that people exhibiting certain types of behaviors ought to be coerced. And we can imagine people holding that mental illness does exist and at the same time holding that some or all of currently practiced psychiatric coercion is unwarranted. Why should the existence of literal mental illness be considered—either by Szasz or by his opponents—as decisive, or even relevant, for the policy issue of psychiatric coercion?

What Szasz Does Not Dispute

Szasz does not dispute the existence of the forms of behavior customarily classified as mental illness (Szasz, 2001, pp. 114–115). He does not deny, for instance, that people sometimes become very sad or anxious for no apparently commensurate reason, or that they sometimes believe very fanciful things, or that their speech and other behavior sometimes takes on baffling nonstandard forms, or that they sometimes seriously injure themselves from what look like bizarre motives. Szasz insists that these are not illnesses or symptoms of illnesses, any more than they are examples of possession by evil spirits. Szasz calls them "problems in living" (Szasz, 1991, p. 19).

Szasz also does not deny the existence of brain conditions, including brain diseases, which affect people's behavior and emotions, sometimes for the worse. Iodine deficiency, syphilis of the brain, epilepsy, head injury, ingestion of toxic substances, Alzheimer's dementia, are some uncontentious examples of medical conditions which may have harmful consequences in people's emotions and behavior. It is uncontroversial that brain conditions may have emotional and behavioral symptoms, or in other words, mental symptoms.

Szasz points out that many of these mental symptoms used to be viewed as purely psychological in origin because the underlying physical conditions of the brain were not known. And when these underlying conditions did become known, these patterns of behavior and feeling were then taken away from psychiatry:

> As soon as a disease thought to be mental is proven to be physical, it is removed from the domain of psychiatry and placed in that of

medicine, to be treated henceforth by internists, neurologists, or neurosurgeons. This is what happened with paresis, pellagra, epilepsy, and brain tumors. (Szasz, 1997, p. 70)

Since Szasz accepts the common-sense medical view that many patterns of behavior and feeling were once observed and discussed (and even treated) without their neurological causes being known, and that these causes were later identified, he has to acknowledge that there are very likely some present-day patterns where the neurological cause is unknown, but where this cause will probably be discovered in the future (Szasz, 1997, 52).

The Metamorphosis of Metaphor

The crucial point disputed by Szasz is not the existence of physical illnesses with mental consequences, but the description of these illnesses as literally mental. In his view, only the body can be literally sick, ill, or diseased. To say that the mind is sick is to employ a metaphor, like saying that the economy is sick or that the condition of the contemporary novel is sick.

Szasz's claim that literal mental illness doesn't exist is, I think, true, with a couple of big qualifications.

The first qualification is that the line between literal and metaphorical is not always sharp. For example, when we set a trap for someone in a poker game, do we view the expression "setting a trap" as literal or metaphorical? This kind of usage no doubt arose as an analogy with preparing a mechanical snare or a concealed pit for an animal (or human) victim, but what was once a metaphor has become so commonplace over many centuries that we hardly think of it as a metaphor. Someone might learn the use of this term in competitive games or in espionage without even knowing about the original meaning.

Or again, the first person to talk about a "virus" that infects a computer was no doubt employing a metaphor, but it's not so clear that it remains a metaphor today. It may be that the use of the word "virus" in the computer context is now so well established that it is no longer a metaphor. If biologists replaced "virus" with a new term and the use of the old term was completely forgotten in its biological context, this might have no effect on the use of the term "virus" in the computer context.

In some cases, a word usage evolves so that people don't even know about the original meaning. Most people who use the expression "plain sailing" don't know that it was once spelled "plane sailing" and referred to the assumption that the surface of the sea was flat rather than curved, which greatly simplified the calculation of a ship's position at the cost of introducing a slight inaccuracy. Here the metaphor has broken completely free of its origins, and people who employ the phrase can hardly be said to be using a metaphor, because they have never known what was once the literal meaning.

It's a matter for judgment whether this has occurred yet with "mental illness." I accept that it has not. However in this case, the more general (or as we would now tend to suppose "metaphorical") usage was the original one. In old-fashioned but still comprehensible expressions like "It's an ill wind that blows no one any good," or "Don't think ill of me," we see the ancient usage of "ill" to apply to anything wrong, unfortunate, or amiss. If English speakers six centuries ago had had any notion of an entity called "the economy," they would have had no hesitation in saying "Something is ill with the economy" or perhaps even "We have an ill economy this year," and they would have meant it literally. Indeed Szasz does say that the modern, scientific meaning of illness or disease, which he contrasts with its metaphorical sense in the phrase "mental illness," is less than two centuries old (Szasz, 2001, pp. 12–15).

The Nonexistence of Literal Mental Illness

Szasz is right to say that mental illness is no literal illness, because the word "illness" in its strictly medical context has acquired a very precise meaning, and this is the only meaning that most people immediately think of when they encounter the word "illness." Furthermore, many proponents of "mental" illness make their nonmetaphorical position more difficult to defend by insisting that mental illness is illness "just like any other illness."

Szasz accepts that there are (or might easily be) as yet unidentified brain diseases with characteristic patterns of emotional and behavioral effects. (From now on, for brevity, I will use the expression "brain diseases with mental symptoms.") It follows that people, such as psychiatrists, might notice the same pattern of mental effects recurring in a number of people, and *surmise* or *conjecture* that these were due to some as yet unidentified brain disease. And they might, in any particular case, be right. Or, of course, they might be wrong.

We see, then, that Szasz and conventional psychiatry are in one respect much closer together than we might think. Both accept that patterns of emotions and behavior may be caused by a brain disease, including the possibility of a brain disease that we haven't identified, and perhaps don't even know how to look for.

So exactly where do Szasz and conventional psychiatry differ? One answer might be that they differ because conventional psychiatrists persist in using the term "mental illness." But Szasz can have no objection to the term "brain disease with mental symptoms," and if, when psychiatrists say "mental illness," they actually mean "brain disease with mental symptoms," then Szasz's objection becomes a somewhat trivial and purely semantic point.

We still speak of "sunrise" and "sunset," even though we know that these terms are literally incorrect. Provided we understand that the sun does not really rise or set, but becomes observable or unobservable because the Earth is spinning, no harm is done by continuing with the traditional terminology, which taken strictly literally might be misleading. Similarly, if psychiatrists say "mental illness" and mean "brain disease with mental symptoms," provided they do understand that minds cannot strictly be sick, there can be no objection that they are mistaking a metaphor for literal truth. They might be making a different mistake, such as thinking there is a brain disease when there really isn't, but they can't be accused of taking a metaphor literally.

So this is my second big qualification. Just as it would be excessively pedantic to object to the word "sunset" in most routine contexts, so it may be excessively pedantic to object to "mental illness," if it is taken to mean "brain disease with mental symptoms." Such an understanding of the phrase seems to be very prevalent today, perhaps more prevalent than ever before. Although the claim that mental illnesses are brain diseases goes back centuries, it is certainly more popular today than fifty years ago. What this development means is that it would not be very difficult for psychiatrists to agree that mental illness is a metaphor and to switch to the term "brain disease with mental symptoms," leaving their other views intact and continuing to favor psychiatric coercion. Szasz does not welcome this trend in psychiatry, but generally tends to give the impression that he dismisses the claim that brain diseases can be attributed to those diagnosed as mentally ill (Szasz, 1997, pp. 49–52, 344–346).

The Virchowian Definition of Disease

If someone observes a pattern of emotion and behavior—what I'm calling a mental pattern—and surmises that these might be caused by a brain disease, Szasz evidently supposes that they are doing something illegitimate. Why would this be illegitimate? The only answer we can extract from Szasz's writings is that this would contradict the Virchowian conception of what qualifies as a disease.

According to this view, associated with Rudolf Virchow (1821–1902), a disease can't be identified unless there is some observable bodily lesion (structural injury or deformity). Thus, nothing can be a disease unless it can be observed by a pathologist. If it can't be identified in a cadaver, it is not a disease. A corpse can have atherosclerosis or bunions, therefore these are diseases. A corpse cannot have bipolar disorder or internet addiction, therefore these are not diseases (Szasz, 1997, pp. 71–73).

Some argue that the Virchowian conception is overly restrictive. A corpse can't have a susceptibility to migraine, for example. (In some cases migraines are caused by something observable in the brain, such as a tumor, but most migraines have no such observable bodily correlate.) But aside from that, there are historical cases where the specific physical correlate of a disease was at first unknown, and later became known. (I use the term "correlate" to avoid taking a position on whether the Virchowian theory holds that the physical lesion is the *cause* of the disease or *is* the disease. Szasz seems to think it is the latter, but it is not clear that this was what Virchow held.)

The physical abnormality does not *become* a disease or the physical correlate of a disease when it is discovered. If it were a disease after discovery, then it must have been a disease before discovery. We therefore have to accept that there can be diseases where the physical correlate is not known. What this means is that we have to bear in mind the distinction between qualifying as a disease by some medical convention and actually being a disease. Virchow's rule is a rule of method for physicians, not a rule of philosophical ontology. It is the adoption of a convention for accrediting diseases, not a claim about the possible existence of diseases. It might conceivably be a good rule for physicians to recognize only such diseases as can be associated with a known lesion, but this cannot alter the fact that there are real diseases which cannot be associated with a known lesion. To suppose otherwise would be to consider that epilepsy *became* a disease only when the responsible brain condition was identified, or that bubonic plague *became* a disease only when the *Yersinia pestis* bacterium was found.

Szasz might want to insist that Virchow's rule is a correct rule of method, and ought to be applied in all cases of putative disease. That would rule out all cases of so-called mental illness—we would not be able to call them "brain diseases with mental symptoms" because Virchow's rule doesn't permit us to call anything a disease until we have identified the specific physical condition which defines the disease. But if we observe a characteristic cluster of symptoms, why shouldn't we conjecture that it is the result of a physical condition, such as a brain illness, even though we can't yet identify that physical condition? There is no good reason why we should not entertain some such hypothesis— which is different, of course, from uncritically taking it to be true once we have thought of it.

Szasz's equivocal interpretation of Virchow runs all through his many statements of his position, sometimes rendering these statements self-contradictory. For example:

> Diseases are demonstrable anatomical or physiological lesions that may occur naturally or be caused by human agents. Although diseases may not be recognized or understood, they "exist." People "have" hypertension or malaria, regardless of whether or not they know it or physicians diagnose it. (Szasz, 2010, p. 276)

The first two sentences contradict each other. If the lesion has to be demonstrable, then people cannot have the disease before the lesion is even suspected. And where is the lesion in hypertension (high blood pressure)? There is no lesion, and pathologists cannot discover hypertension in a corpse.

The Virchowian definition does not really help Szasz make his case. Szasz has not come up with some reasoning which prevents us from saying: "We observe certain emotional and behavioral peculiarities. We conjecture that they are symptoms of a disease, whose physical nature has yet to be discovered." No argument has been offered to show that such a way of thinking is illegitimate or wrong-headed.

The conclusion we have arrived at (a conclusion Szasz occasionally seem to dispute but at other times seems to accept, and a conclusion which is in any case practically indisputable) is that there is not necessarily anything wrong with observing mental symptoms, and conjecturing that these might be caused by, and therefore might be symptoms of, a brain condition. This conclusion doesn't mean that any such conjectured condition has actually been accurately specified for any of the currently accepted "mental illnesses." It merely means that no such conjecture can be ruled out a priori. It is up to psychiatrists or others to make a case for the existence of each putative brain disease.

However, the general possibility that there might be as yet unidentified brain diseases with mental symptoms is hardly outlandish, because, for example, we know that intake of some drugs or toxic substances can cause mental symptoms—such as hallucinations, unusual euphoria, intense fearfulness, or difficulty in concentrating one's thoughts—and if such mental symptoms can be caused by ingested chemicals, it is no great leap to suppose that they might also be sometimes caused by other physical changes in the body.

Szasz's Denials of Factual Propositions about Brain Diseases

When discussing various putative psychiatric illnesses—notably schizophrenia, about which Szasz has written more than any other alleged psychiatric disease—Szasz alternates between denying that there is an "it" there at all—that some definite pattern of mental features has been identified—and accepting that there is an "it" while denying that it represents a disease. This alternation can perhaps be defended by saying that Szasz wants to test out both claims of psychiatry independently.

Szasz makes some substantive factual claims about the possibility of brain diseases, which do not follow from his basic insight into the metaphorical nature of mental illness. The crucial point here (for my argument) is not whether Szasz is right or wrong in these claims, but the fact that these claims cannot be logically derived from his fundamental claim about mental illness.

Many psychiatrists now say that various mental illnesses, such as schizophrenia or bipolar disorder, are caused by a chemical imbalance in the brain. Szasz points out that no one has ever observed or detected any such supposed chemical imbalance, which is correct (Valenstein, 1998; Wyatt & Midkiff, 2006, 2007), and well worth bearing in mind, but not relevant to the main point, which is that a chemical imbalance in the brain is one hypothesis to account for a pattern of mental manifestations, and there can be no reason to dismiss this hypothesis out of hand.

Szasz not only states that this supposed chemical imbalance has not been detected, which is true, but also on occasion seems to be implying that there is no such chemical imbalance accounting for, say, schizophrenia. Often, however, we find on close examination of his text that he literally asserts only that there is no *proven* chemical imbalance (1997, pp. 346–349), which is merely another way of saying that the supposed chemical imbalance has not been detected. So what of the possibility that there might be a suspected or conjectured chemical imbalance, which might be a good working hypothesis because other explanations for the observed mental patterns seem inadequate? It is just here that the debate should be focused, but Szasz's approach tends to ignore it.

Szasz's evident claim that there is no chemical imbalance (not just that there is no proven chemical imbalance), emerges most clearly in aphoristic passages like the following:

> If you believe that you are Jesus or that the Communists are after you (and they are not)—then your belief is likely to be regarded as a symptom of schizophrenia. But if you believe that Jesus is the Son of God or that Communism is the only scientifically and morally correct form of government—then your belief is likely to be regarded as a reflection of who you are: Christian or Communist. That is why I think that we will discover the chemical cause of schizophrenia when we discover the chemical cause of Christianity and Communism. No sooner and no later. (Szasz, 1990, pp. 215–216)

The reasoning here seems to be that if one belief is caused by a chemical imbalance, then so must another belief be similarly caused. Now, we know that if you're a Christian or a Communist, you most likely became an adherent of one or another of these doctrinal systems because you were persuaded, as a result of hearing people talk about them, that their essential propositions are true. That's how we know that you did *not* become a Christian or a Communist because of a chemical imbalance in your brain. In contrast, if you came to believe that you are Jesus or that the Communists are after you, this was not because of anyone trying to persuade you of these beliefs. Your adoption of such beliefs showed more originality and independence of thought than the typical Christian or Communist. If it's possible for any beliefs to be the result of chemical imbalances in the brain, the beliefs that you are Jesus or that the Communists are after you do indeed look like better candidates for such causation.

Just to be clear, I suppose we all take it for granted—Szasz evidently did (Szasz, 2010, p. 101)—that if you are a Christian or a Communist this will have some consequences for events going on in your brain. (Because it is not necessary in this context, I do not here explore the question of whether being a Christian or a Communist *is* a matter of events going on in your brain, though that is what I believe.) But in complex systems there can be explanations at different levels, and there can be "downward causation" from higher levels to lower levels, as well as "upward causation" from lower levels to higher (Campbell, 1974; Campbell, 1990). Szasz's assumption of the equivalent causation of different beliefs is not as self-evident as he supposed. It is not entirely preposterous that there could be a chemical-imbalance explanation of paranoid thought-patterns and no chemical-imbalance explanation for the adoption of conventional belief-systems.

Szasz's Non-Sequitur

Because of the eloquent, pithy, and somewhat oracular manner in which Szasz often presents his argument, there is a tendency for readers to suppose that if literal mental illness is an incoherent notion, then schizophrenia cannot be caused by a chemical imbalance. But Szasz doesn't produce any argument to this effect. There is actually no logical connection at all between these two assertions. The hypothetical causation of schizophrenia by a chemical imbalance may turn out to be true or false. (Since decades of research, generously assisted by the pharmaceutical companies, have so far failed to find it, we may be inclined to speculate that its long-term chances, as a scientific hypothesis, do not look promising). But it is not disallowed by the contention that there are no literal mental illnesses. Szasz might be right on both counts, but his second claim is not derivable from his first, and needs to be investigated, tested, and evaluated with different arguments, which must be mainly empirical rather than semantic or conceptual.

Consider this typical assertion by Szasz:

> If we accept the proposition that X is not an illness unless there are *defining, objective, anatomical criteria for it,* in other words, that X is not an illness unless it can be diagnosed by examining some part of the patient's body, then it is absurd to call a condition that lacks precisely that characteristic a "real illness." (Szasz, 2001, p. 83; emphasis in original)

Szasz is forgetting that we already know that "the proposition" must be false, because we know that people have had illnesses before anyone had found their anatomical criteria. Leave aside the point that not everyone agrees with that definition of an illness—some people would say that a person who experiences migraine attacks actually has an illness. Still, we recall that Szasz himself accepts that people throughout history were really ill long before the "defining, objective, anatomical criteria" of their illnesses were discovered. The absurdity Szasz points to does not arise if someone says: "I admit that we can't yet establish the anatomical signs of this illness, but I conjecture that there is such an illness."

This thought naturally occurred to Szasz, who, immediately after the above, writes "It may happen in medicine that we do not yet know whether a problematic condition is or is not illness" (tacitly conceding again that X may be an illness when we have no anatomical criteria for it). He goes on to say that in criminal justice, it is considered better to let a thousand guilty persons go free than to convict a single innocent person, whereas "our medical maxim is that it is better to falsely diagnose and unnecessarily treat a thousand healthy persons than to mistakenly declare a single sick person healthy and thus deprive him of treatment."

Here Szasz has quietly dropped his immediately preceding claim of absurdity. It may be mistaken policy, it may even be an appalling scandal, to treat a thousand people unnecessarily to be sure of helping the one who really benefits from treatment, but there's nothing absurd about it. The problem in Szasz's presentation of his argument arises from his tendency not to make a sharp distinction between someone actually having an illness and that person's complying with the practical requirement we may have adopted to recognize him as having an accredited illness.

Where did Szasz get the thousand-to-one ratio from? In the immediate context of Szasz's remarks we can infer that if a person or his family insist that there is something wrong with him, and medical tests can discover nothing wrong with him, Szasz says that under current arrangements he will always be "given treatment" for a "mental illness," and Szasz's estimate of the likelihood that he will actually have something medically wrong with him is one in a thousand-and-one.

Szasz's position, then, is that people see psychiatrists because of problems they have or problems other people have with them. These problems may possibly be due to brain diseases which have not yet been physically identified, but this (in Szasz's judgment) can only be true in a tiny minority of cases at most. Szasz assumes that the great majority of people (picturesquely, one thousand out of every 1,001) who see psychiatrists don't have any unidentified brain disease. What this amounts to is the proposition that "mental illnesses" (brain diseases with mental symptoms) are at the very least hugely overdiagnosed. This may well be true (I think it very likely is) but it has no logical relation to the claim that there are no literal mental illnesses.

Many psychiatrists and other mental health professionals talk as if all problems in living are diseases. Notice, however, that there is a distinction between the claim that some apparent problems in living, referred to by psychiatry as diseases, are not diseases—that there is an area of human behavior, choice, emotion, and suffering which does not belong to the domain of psychiatry or medicine—and the claim that all such problems in living are not diseases (or caused by diseases). The first claim, one with which I agree, makes up the topic of much of Szasz's writing—his trenchant and witty exposure of the follies of mental-health imperialism. As to the second claim, I'm more inclined to doubt it. But in any case, the two claims are not the same claim.

In correspondence with Szasz about *The Myth of Mental Illness*, Sir Karl Popper stated that he believed Szasz was "95% right" but did not accept the total nonexistence of mental illness. The published extracts from the correspondence (Schaler, 2004, p. 136) do not make absolutely clear what Popper meant here, but I think it's reasonable to surmise that he meant that something like 95 percent of what is labeled mental illness is no illness at all, as Szasz maintained, whereas the other 5 percent of it is (contrary to Szasz) due to brain disease. My impression is that this is what a lot of thoughtful people, dubious about the pretensions of psychiatric imperialism, do believe. Naturally, there's no significance in the precise figure of 5 percent. It might be 1 percent or it might be 20 percent.

Psychiatry has moved both closer to Szasz's position and further away from it. Fifty years ago, psychiatrists would be more likely to adhere to psychoanalytic notions of the causation of mental diseases/problems in living. Now they are more likely to insist that such problems must be due to a purely physical cause, such as chemical imbalance in the brain. This is closer to Szasz's position in that it harmonizes better with the view that if something is a disease, it can only be a disease of the body. But it is further away from Szasz's position because it views as medical problems states of affairs which in his judgment we should not regard as medical at all. The early Szasz was decidedly an adherent of psychoanalysis in its then fashionable incarnations of ego psychology, object-relations theory, and interpersonal psychology (Szasz, 2010, pp. 95–101, 213–225). The later Szasz no longer expressed any support for psychoanalytic theory, and perhaps had become disillusioned with it. But Szasz always held that people with problems in living can be helped by psychotherapy, which consists in talking with them about their subjective mental life—including their assumptions, goals, and values. And psychotherapy falls within a liberal definition of "psychoanalysis." From Szasz's point of view, psychoanalysis, broadly defined, was at least attempting to treat people as human beings, while the medical approach tends to dehumanize them by converting their real personal and ethical problems into diseases. However, this stance ignores the question: are some of these people's real human problems due to disorders of their brains? As we have seen, despite superficial appearance, Szasz has never offered us any reason to discount this possibility a priori.

Consider Szasz's famous and moving essay, "What Psychiatry Can and Cannot Do" (Szasz, 1991, pp. 79–86). In the first page or two, Szasz briefly mentions and criticizes the concept of mental illness. Then, he presents a number of pseudonymous case histories which display, in heart-rending fashion, the disgraceful horrors routinely perpetrated by modern psychiatry. However, these case histories would be just as effective in calling psychiatric practice into question if they were not preceded by his dismissive mention of "mental illness." We could delete the reference to mental illness, and then a believer in the existence of some brain diseases with mental symptoms could easily respond to these case histories by saying, "Yes, isn't it sad the damage psychiatry can do when it becomes corrupt and is allowed to stray outside its proper area of competence? We should be much more careful about defining the area in which psychiatry can operate, and repudiating its pretensions outside this circumscribed area."

Although he often seems to be rejecting the possibility that mental symptoms might be due to an as yet unidentified brain disease, Szasz also expresses the view that it would make little or no difference if brain correlates for putative diseases such as schizophrenia were to be discovered (1990, pp. 222–224). And he has also asserted that such a discovery would actually strengthen his own argument against coercive psychiatry (Szasz, 1997, p. 347).

What Would Justify Psychiatric Coercion?

Szasz has given us no reason to rule out a priori the possibility that we can conjecture, from observing someone's behavior, that they have a brain disease with mental symptoms, though we don't yet know (and may never know) what physical condition in their brain constitutes the disease.

The fact that this conjecture makes sense and can't be ruled out doesn't imply that any claim as to the existence of any such brain disease is true. What would incline us to suppose it might be true in any particular instance?

First, we would need clear evidence that there is an "it" there at all. What this means in practice is that if a large number of psychiatrists were to "examine" (talk to) a person, a very high percentage of them (close to 100 percent) should agree on whether this person has or does

97

not have a mental illness (a brain disease with mental symptoms), and if so, precisely what that mental illness is. We expect this from doctors deciding whether someone has cancer or atherosclerosis, and we expect something analogous from accountants auditing a company's financial records. We should certainly never take these opinions very seriously if we think there is frequent disagreement on actual cases among these accredited experts.

It is particularly important to insist on this minimum condition because there are no physical tests for these hypothesized brain diseases. The supposed diseases are only surmised to account for the patient's behavior or mental state. There has never been a case, and with current knowledge never could be a case, where the psychiatrist says to the patient: "The test results have come back from the lab and I'm happy to inform you that you do not have schizophrenia." (Or: "Your family say you're an asshole, but unfortunately for them, science says you're a sane asshole.") There are no lab tests for schizophrenia or depression, and if in the future such tests were ever to be developed, these conditions would, as Szasz often reminds us, become recognized as neurological diseases, not the province of psychiatry.

Unanimity or near-unanimity of diagnosis by numerous psychiatrists of the same patient would be an essential requirement for allowing the hypothesis that the patient has a brain disease to affect policy, but it would still not prove that he had a brain disease. People's behavior often falls into regularly recurring patterns for reasons other than that they all have a chemical imbalance in their brains. It might be that the psychiatrists are indeed detecting a common pattern—that there really is an "it" there—but that this pattern is not due to a brain disease. So before we accepted that a person's behavior were accounted for by a brain disease, we would have to see arguments, based on the peculiar nature of his particular behavior, that it was not better explained by some alternative hypothesis.

Suppose then, that the cluster of symptoms is unanimously identified and that alternative explanations don't look very convincing. In a particular instance, we decide that a good case has been made that we're dealing with a brain disease. This is still a long way from justifying coercion. If we look at those brain diseases where the physical cause in the brain has actually been found—epilepsy, Alzheimer's, or stroke—the sufferers are not normally locked up and no one thinks they should be. Contrary to Virchow's rule, I think that migraine (or susceptibility to migraine) is obviously a brain disease where the brain defect has not (in most cases) been discovered. And yet no one thinks migraine sufferers should be locked up. In fact, there is no legal provision for committing anyone with a known brain disease, and the moment a physical cause for schizophrenia were established, the immediate effect might be that schizophrenics *qua* schizophrenics could not be committed. Judges or juries routinely commit or acquit people on the basis of testimony by psychiatrists, almost never on the basis of testimony by neurologists. To save the situation (and an important portion of their income) psychiatrists would probably maintain that these patients had something wrong with them in addition to the newly identified brain condition, something which, in turn, would be attributed to an additional and still-unknown brain condition. This response becomes even more likely because the newly discovered physical cause for schizophrenia would almost certainly not apply to some diagnosed cases of schizophrenia, and a way would have to be found for continuing to deprive those patients of their normal legal protections.

The general rule of the medical profession is that individuals may not be treated against their will, no matter how imperative this may seem to the physician and no matter how foolish the individual may be in refusing treatment. This holds just as much for brain disease as for lung disease.

Two reasons are suggested for why "the mentally ill" should be consigned to a mental hospital against their wishes. One is that they are dangerous to the public or to themselves. Another is that due to their disease, their judgment is impaired, so that they cannot seek the treatment they would seek if their judgment were not impaired—a veritable Catch-22.

Both these rationales for coercion are, on the face of it, not overwhelmingly convincing. Do people diagnosed as schizophrenic or bipolar attack other people more frequently than random members of the general population? And if they do, do they do so by a greater percentage than Ethnic Group A, Religious Group X, or Occupational Group Q (take your choice)?

In practice, most discussion of involuntary commitment could easily be detached from any psychiatric input. If someone says "Charles Manson should be locked up for life," this has obvious common-sense appeal, whether we think that Manson is a schizophrenic (and schizophrenia is a brain disease), a schizophrenic (and schizophrenia is not a brain disease), a demon, a human possessed by a demon, a vampire, a zombie, a golem, a space alien, or a very wicked person with fanciful beliefs. Psychiatrists do not know of any technique which could reliably convert Manson into a competent yet nonthreatening individual. So the only serious practical question here is whether the public can be protected from Manson by methods which do not contravene the rights and liberties Manson has in common with everyone else.

Next consider the notion that someone cannot be allowed to choose whether he will have treatment or not, because he suffers from a brain disease that impairs his judgment.

The mere fact that someone's judgment is not very good is not normally considered sufficient to justify their coercive treatment. Many individuals not diagnosed as mentally ill may show poor judgment, while many individuals diagnosed as mentally ill may show excellent judgment. Poor judgment comes with the territory of being human, and individuals must to some extent take the consequences of their poor judgment. We don't, for example, coercively set aside a person's decision to seek a divorce, sell their house, buy a car, donate organs to medical research, join the Moonies, raise all-in on the flop, or make a will, merely because their judgment is poor. (They may be ruled incompetent, but that is generally a matter of whether they understand what's going on, something in principle distinct from any diagnosis of brain disease.) In all walks of life except psychiatry, we acknowledge that individuals are perfectly entitled to act upon their poor judgment. Someone who "hears voices" may be distracted, and may therefore make poor decisions, but so may someone else be distracted by a painful back condition, rowdy neighbors, or a spouse's nagging.

All kinds of "mentally ill" people do voluntarily seek treatment, so it cannot be a general rule that a symptom of some mental illness is unwillingness to be treated. Persons with no diagnosis of mental illness often decline to seek treatment for a disease, and physicians cannot compel them, no matter how strongly they feel that these persons are being foolish.

As a background to this discussion, there is the research material indicating that people classified as seriously mentally ill can in general be relied upon to make rational choices. Studies of the most hopeless cases of psychosis show that the psychotics act rationally: they respond to incentives. Given rewards for behaving in particular ways, they adapt their behavior to comply (Battalio et al., 1973; Winkler, 1970, 1972). The same applies to addicts (addiction is still often labeled a mental illness): studies invariably show that even the most hardened and recalcitrant addicts will adjust their drug consumption. For example, the most hopeless institutionalized cases of extreme alcoholism, if given free access to alcohol along with rewards for moderating their alcohol consumption, will moderate. There is similar evidence for conscious control exercised by heroin and cocaine addicts (Schaler, 2000, pp. 21–32).

The usual joke here is that "they may be crazy but they're not stupid." However, nonstupidity sets a limit to craziness. People diagnosed as seriously mentally ill generally make intelligible choices. As for always making the best choices, that's not something we're entitled to demand of any group of people on pain of their being incarcerated without trial.

Szasz has attacked psychiatry on many different grounds. Some of these grounds are effective, quite independently of his pedantic denial of the literal existence of mental illness, and may even lose some of their impact by being associated with it.

One of the most persuasive reasons offered by Szasz for viewing psychiatric theory as a pseudoscience is that it changes its diagnostic categories by a process of political horse-trading among interest groups and advocacy groups. Some examples are well-known. Until 1973, American psychiatry classified homosexuality as a disease. Since 1973, homosexuality has not been a disease. This switch was not indicated by any research or any theoretical developments. No findings had been published with the remotest bearing on the question of whether homosexuality is a disease. The switch was made in response to pressure from gay rights groups. When an APA "working group" was revising the DSM and proposing to identify rape (or "rapism") as a mental disease, feminists were concerned that this diagnosis might get rapists off, so the psychiatrists caved to the feminists. They similarly abandoned the labeling as "masochism" of women who remain in abusive relationships (Szasz, 1997, pp. 79–80).

What are we to make of this? Obviously, that the theory of psychiatry is largely pseudoscience, not genuine science, and certainly not a genuine branch of medicine. No other branch of medicine would behave like this; it would be a scandal if they did. Yet we have no guarantee that even pseudoscience may not stumble upon the truth in particular instances. So again, we cannot conclude that there is no such thing as an unidentified brain disease with mental symptoms, just because this forms part of a currently thriving pseudoscience.

Szasz and the Mind–Body Problem

Why did Szasz lay such emphasis on the mythical nature of mental illness, and continue to do so over the decades, leading to widespread misunderstanding of his arguments against coercive psychiatry? I

101

don't know the answer, but I suspect that it is related to an odd feature of Szasz's thinking—his unsatisfactory conception of the relation between mind and brain. It is, at the very least, clear that events in the mind can affect events in the brain and vice versa, and so we would expect someone who has spent a lifetime discussing mental illness, with a large part of that concerned with the possibility that what is called mental illness is due to brain disease, to take a position on the relation of mind and brain, or at least to disclose some interesting views on the topic.

To consider such matters as the causation of mental symptoms by brain diseases, it helps to have some conception of what philosophers traditionally call the mind–body problem, which given modern knowledge of the brain, means the relation between mind and brain. This relation between mind and brain is an area where Szasz seems to have very definite views, and yet simultaneously is strangely reticent.

As we read most of Szasz's work, we become conscious of an odd lacuna: he repeatedly draws a bright line between consciousness and physiology, as though these are independent realms. He discusses mental events as though they generally happen independently of brain events. This is the more remarkable because he is an atheist with no theological commitments. We wonder what he thinks about the relation of mind and brain. With *The Meaning of Mind*, (1996) we find out that he has no coherent view of the relation between mind and brain and (while the book does have a sprinkling of keen insights here and there) his uninformed comments on those who have carefully elaborated various philosophical theories often miss the point.

Szasz briskly reviews a number of writers, whom he presents as adherents of a "new cult" (Szasz, 1996, p. 81) he calls "neurophilosophy"—Daniel Dennett, Patricia Churchland, Paul Churchland, John Searle, Karl Popper and John Eccles, Francis Crick, and Julian Jaynes. If he had merely pointed out that some of these (such as the Churchlands) have erroneous beliefs about psychiatry, Szasz would have been on safer ground. He pays almost no attention to the differences between these thinkers. It is hard to imagine philosophers more different in their fundamental mind–body theories than Dennett, Searle, and Popper, and it would be helpful to know what Szasz thought about these differences, but Szasz writes as though he knows nothing of them. Some of Szasz's remarks seem to suggest he would be closest to Popper's interactionism, but he is so determinedly reticent on the mind–body relation that we can't be sure. Jaynes is a psychologist and popular writer whom almost all philosophers would dismiss as a fanciful proponent of a demonstrably false historical thesis.

What seems to concern Szasz is that all the writers he mentions here acknowledge a close association of mind and brain, and even go so far as to equate the two. He fastens on this aspect of their thinking (usually just turning up a quotation where they assert the equivalence of mind and brain) and does not pursue any other aspect of their thinking. Szasz attributes the denial of personal responsibility to all of those mentioned (p. 76), dubious in several cases and an egregious blunder when applied to Searle or Popper (Searle, 2007; Popper, 1972). His unfamiliarity with the area is indicated by his not knowing that "intentionality" has a specialized meaning in philosophy of mind—he assumes it refers to intentions (p. 82).

I can find no more than three things we can be sure of in Szasz's view of the mind–brain relation: that the mind cannot exist without the body (Szasz, 1996, p. 76) (agreed by almost everyone); that the mind is not the brain; and that the mind is not defined by consciousness (Szasz, 1996, p. 81). Szasz thinks that mind and brain cannot be the same because we have two different words for them (p. 75) which likewise show that the Morning Star is not the Evening Star and that heat is not molecular motion. Szasz maintains that "equating mind with brain implies a denial of the distinctively human activities called 'minding,' 'talking to oneself,' and 'being responsible'" (p. 75), but offers no reason for this claim, which most of the writers he is discussing would reject. (I take it for granted that the equivalence of mind and brain is a kind of hyperbole, if only because the brain controls autonomic functions like heartbeat which are not part of the mind. A stricter formulation would be that the mind consists of a class of brain events.)

A general theme of Szasz's remarks here (75–80) is that persons are not brains and that no "materialist account" can be given of persons. But then, where is the person located? It has to be: 1. the brain; 2. some other part of the body; 3. somewhere other than the body; or 4. nowhere at all. Which? Szasz doesn't give us any hint as to what his answer would be. It seems clear to me that the person is inside the skull, but I accept that there are other views which can be defended. When it comes to the relation of mind and brain as a philosophical topic, Szasz does not offer us anything which would help us understand his conception of the mind–brain relation.

In Conclusion

Szasz advances two claims, which he evidently supposes are tightly connected. These claims are that there is no such thing as literal mental illness and that psychiatric coercion is wrong. These claims may both be correct (I think they are), but they are not tightly connected. Szasz's denial of the literal existence of mental illness is an interesting conceptual insight, but contrary to his own apparent view, it has few implications for policy.

Szasz has developed some effective arguments against psychiatric coercion, and against the pretensions of psychiatry generally, but these arguments are strictly independent of his conceptual thesis about mental illness, and might have been more persuasive if they had been elaborated without the distraction of that conceptual analysis.

If I am right, then arguing that there is no literal mental illness is neither necessary nor particularly effective in making a case against psychiatric coercion. It's quite correct as a piece of conceptual analysis— "a mind diseased" is indeed an incoherent notion, as the doctor hinted (but was too tactful to state explicitly) in response to Macbeth (*Macbeth*, Act V, Scene 3). There can literally be no such thing as a mental illness. But this is a pedantic point, like the literal nonexistence of sunrise and sunset.

Today the most popular unpacking of "mental illness" by far is "unidentified brain illness with mental symptoms," and there is nothing incoherent about that. Attempts to deny outright that such things exist are misplaced, because there is every reason to surmise that such things could exist. On the other hand, psychiatry's claims to have identified such entities, constructed from mental symptoms alone, are often dubious in particular cases, and even the definite acceptance of such psychiatric diagnoses would not take us very far toward justifying psychiatric coercion.

Critics of psychiatric theory and psychiatric coercion should not lay too much emphasis on the literal nonexistence of mental illness, but should do what Szasz in fact did much of the time: criticize both the foundations of specific psychiatric diagnoses and the arguments for withholding from those diagnosed as "mentally ill" the usual civil liberties and legal protections enjoyed by all other competent adults.

References

Battalio, R.C., Kagel, J. H., Winkler, R. C., Fisher, Jr. E. B., Basmann, R. L., & Krasner, L. (1973). A test of consumer demand theory using observations of individual consumer purchases. *Economic Inquiry, 11*, 4.

Campbell, D. T. (1974). Downward causation in hierarchically organised biological systems. In Francisco Jose Ayala & Theodosius Dobzhansky (Eds.), *Studies in the philosophy of biology: Reduction and related problems*. London: Macmillan.

Campbell, D. T. (1990). Levels of organization, downward causation, and the selection-theory approach to evolutionary epistemology. In Gary Greenberg & Ethel Tobach (Eds.), *Theories of the evolution of knowing*. Hillsdale: Erlbaum.

Popper, K. R. (1972). *Objective knowledge: An evolutionary approach*. Oxford: Oxford University Press.

Schaler, J. A. (2000). *Addiction is a choice*. Chicago: Open Court.

Schaler, Jeffrey A. (ed.). 2004. *Szasz under fire: The psychiatric abolitionist faces his critics*. Chicago: Open Court.

Searle, J. R. (2007). *Freedom and neurobiology: Reflections on free will, language, and political power*. New York: Columbia University Press.

Szasz, T. S. (1960). The myth of mental illness. *American Psychologist, 15*, 113.

Szasz, T. S. (1976). *Schizophrenia: The sacred symbol of psychiatry*. New York: Basic Books.

Szasz, T. S. (1990). *The untamed tongue: A dissenting dictionary*. La Salle: Open Court.

Szasz, T. S. (1991) [1970]. *Ideology and insanity: Essays on the psychiatric dehumanization of man*. Syracuse: Syracuse University Press.

Szasz, T. S. (1997) [1987]. *Insanity: The idea and its consequences*. Syracuse: Syracuse University Press.

Szasz, T. S. (2001). *Pharmacracy: Medicine and politics in America*. Westport: Praeger.

Szasz, T. S. (2002) [1996]. *The meaning of mind: Language, morality, and neuroscience*. Syracuse: Syracuse University Press.

Szasz, T. S. (2007). *The medicalization of everyday life: Selected essays*. Syracuse: Syracuse University Press.

Szasz, T. S. (2010) [1961]. *The myth of mental illness: Foundations of a theory of personal conduct*. New York: Harper Perennial.

Valenstein, E. S. (1998). *Blaming the brain: The truth about drugs and mental health*. New York: The Free Press.

Winkler, R. C. (1970). Management of chronic psychiatric patients by a token reinforcement system. *Journal of Applied Behavior Analysis, 3* (Spring), 47–55.

Winkler, R. C. (1972). An experimental analysis of economic balance: Savings and wages in a token economy. *Behavior Therapy, 4*, 1.

Wyatt, W. J., & Midkiff, D. M. (2006). Biological psychiatry: A practice in search of a science. *Behavior and Social Issues, 15*, 132–151.

Wyatt, W. J., & Midkiff, D. M. (2007). Psychiatry's thirty-five-year, non-empirical reach for biological explanations. *Behavior and Social Issues, 16*, 197–213.

Part III

Through a Szaszian Lens

6

"False Truths" about Addiction: Thomas Szasz and Karl Polanyi

Bruce K. Alexander

As he grew up in Europe amidst an outbreak of fascism that eventually precipitated World War II, Thomas Szasz came face-to-face with the "invincible social power of false truths" (Szasz, 2004a, p. 27). Along with the racial and authoritarian "false truths" of the day, he saw that tyrannical regimes sometimes labeled deviations from their norms as "mental illnesses" so that doctors could "cure" them by coercive and often harmful medical interventions.

Szasz and his Jewish family escaped the growing fascist threat in Europe just in time. Thomas and his brother George emigrated to the United States in 1938. Tragically, however, the young Thomas Szasz soon caught the scent of tyranny again in his new home. Szasz's suspicion that the concept of mental illness was being used for tyrannical purposes deepened during his American training in medicine, psychiatry, and psychoanalysis and as he encountered unsettling contradictions in American culture (Szasz, 1970, 1973/1985, 2004a, pp. 18–28). Szasz's youthful suspicions have now been borne out in many domains.

Addiction

Szasz's multipronged critique of the concept of mental illness has proven particularly applicable to the field of addiction.

Recent research has confirmed much of what Szasz claimed about addiction in his book *Ceremonial Chemistry* (Szasz, 1973/1985). As Szasz argued, classifying any kind of addiction as either a sin or a disease is both scientifically dubious and easily blended into the tyranny

In the discussion that follows, I have avoided all medicalized defini-tions of the word "addiction." I have consistently used the word "addic-tion" in its normal sense in the English language, that is, definition 1a of the unabridged *Oxford English Dictionary* (2010 edition).

> 1a. The state or condition of being dedicated or devoted to a thing, esp. an activity or occupation; adherence or attachment, esp. of an immoderate or compulsive kind . . .

This is the way the word was used by Shakespeare, the King James Version of the Bible, David Hume, Charles Dickens, and other masters of the English language. Outside of the medicalized field of addiction, it has been the primary definition up to the present day. Please take note that this traditional definition does not define addiction in terms of *either* sin *or* disease; that it does not limit addiction to alcohol and drugs; and that it encompasses the full range of severity from mild and inconsequential to severe and dangerous. The traditional definition is hard to operationalize, but the incidence of addiction thus defined can be studied historically and linguistically, especially since the invention of the Google Ngram Viewer (Google Books, undated).

Today's society is concerned with severe, dangerous forms of addiction to drug use and a great variety of other pursuits that last for extended periods and do harm to individual addicted people and to society. These addictions are a *subset* of the domain of the traditional definition. When referring to this subset of addictions in this chap-ter, I have consistently used the term "severe addiction." Like the full traditional definition, "severe addiction" is a way of living that is not defined in terms of moral failure, disease, alcohol, or drugs. There are many ways of operationalizing "severe addiction" for use in quanti-tative interview research (Alexander & Schweighofer, 1988; Case & Deaton, 2015).

of the War on Drugs as well as the oppressive practices of what Szasz called "Institutional Psychiatry" and the "Therapeutic State" (Peele, 1989; Schaler, 2000; Pearson, 2004; Pickard, 2012; Ahmed et al., 2013; Levy, 2013; Satel & Lilienfeld, 2013; Hall et al., 2014; Alexander, 2014).

History also confirms Szasz's claim that medical treatment of severe addiction has much in common with the witch-hunts and inquisitions of past centuries. Much of the "treatment" that supposedly drug-addicted people have received is futile and some is punitive. Drug addicts have served as scapegoats for all of society's ills. Many of the people subjected to involuntary treatment for severe addiction could not be called "addicted," by any reasonable definition of the word (e.g., Roth, 1964; Peele, 1989; Hari, 2015).

Yet the medical interpretation of severe addiction maintains a near official status in government and institutionalized medicine, although current versions are stated in nonpunitive language. The medical model of severe addiction is widely accepted by scientists and the public today (Alexander, 2014; *Nature* editorial, 2014; Seelye, 2015). In the field of addiction, Szasz's lament over the "the invincible social power of false truths" still rings true.

Whereas Szasz's critique of the medicalization of severe addiction has proven correct, his alternative explanations for the lifestyles that are being medically diagnosed as addiction have not held up as well. It is *not* enough to say, as Szasz did in various places, that drug addicted people just "like to use drugs" or that addiction is "a problem in living"; a "ceremonial practice"; a "self medication" for physical disease; a yielding to temptation; or a useful habit that people pursue of their "own free will" and abandon if it becomes counterproductive. Although these formulations do describe many drug users and mildly addicted people, they do not address the misery and hopelessness that grows from severe addictions.

Severe addiction has been spreading over the globe in an ever deeper and wider flood throughout the late modern era (Alexander, 2008/2010). Not only are severe addictions to alcohol and drugs still on the rise in the twenty-first century (see Case & Deaton, 2015, Fig. 4; Munro, 2015), but there are also very large numbers of severe "process addictions" or "behavioral addictions," where drugs do not play a major role (Sussman et al., 2010).

Szasz seemed to shrug off the current flood of severe addictions by treating it either as a fad of pathological self-definition or as a side effect of the medicalization and prohibition of drug use (Szasz, 1970, pp. 38–40, 1973/1985, p. xiii, 4, 11–12, 170–171). More recent writers have advanced similar ideas (Cohen, 2000; Frances, 2013, pp. 88–92). However, this easy dismissal fits with neither the experience of severely addicted people nor with the history of addiction.

Despite the fact that severely addicted people are not "ill" in any useful sense of the word, many do suffer terribly, and often die in misery. Many of them seriously harm themselves, their families, their society, and the planet Earth (Alexander, 2015; Case & Deaton, 2015).

Although many people are severely addicted to alcohol or drugs, more are likely to be severely addicted to gambling, food, internet games, exercise, social media, sex, love, wealth, shopping, power, fashions, celebrity worship, cult practices, etc. Moreover, the prevalence of severe addiction is not a historical constant. It varies from an almost indetectable minority of the population in some times and places to an apparent majority in others, including our own (Alexander, 2008/2010; Sussman et al., 2010). This is much more than what Szasz called the "so-called 'problem' . . . of drug addiction" (1973/1985, p. 4) that can be easily shrugged off.

The question of why there are huge numbers of severely addicted people in the late modern era has not been adequately answered by Szasz, nor by the army of addiction experts who have preceded and followed him. But why not?

I believe that the question has not been answered because almost all the questioners, including Szasz himself, have assumed that addiction is an *individual* problem. On the contrary, I believe that it is a *societal* problem that is built into the social, political, and economic structure of the modern era as well as some eras in the past (Alexander, 2008/2010; Alexander & Shelton, 2014, chap. 4). I believe that severe addiction is as inseparable from life in the modern world as competitiveness, anxiety, depression, and wasteful consumption. That is why it is not possible to solve the widespread addiction problem by punishment of individuals (as Szasz showed), or by forced treatment of individuals (as Szasz showed), *or* by greater assertion of individual will power (although Szasz seemed to think it might be) or by ignoring its existence, as Szasz was wont to do. (See Szasz, 1970, pp. 38–40, 1973/1985, p. xiii, 4, 11–12).

If I am right, the biggest "false truth" in the addiction field today is the widespread assumption that severe addiction is an individual, rather than a societal problem. The greatest irony is that Szasz, an intrepid slayer of other false truths, accepted the biggest false truth about severe addiction himself. The biggest challenge is that addiction can only be brought under control by changing the structure of modern society.

The biggest tribute to the legacy of Thomas Szasz that I can imagine would be to emulate his indomitable courage by exposing a "false truth" that is as important as those that he himself exposed, although I will limit mine to the subfield of addiction, rather than taking on the whole field of mental health, as he did. Of course, those of us who make it our business to reveal false truths in the field of addiction can only hope to succeed because Szasz, and other pioneers, broke the trail. The critical task that they began is still underway, even though one of its most renowned trailbreakers has now taken his turn to rest.

Thomas Szasz and Karl Polanyi: Across a Political Chasm

Thomas Szasz conceptualized the problem of addiction in a twentieth-century context of menacing nation states and embattled individuals. As an atheistic, Hungarian Jew he had experienced intolerance at first hand and believed it was his personal duty to resist it (Szasz, 2004b, 1973/1985, p. 87).

From Szasz's libertarian viewpoint, deviance, possibly including drug use, was essential for individuals who hoped to create an intellectual, artistic, or entrepreneurial place in the world. This standpoint inspired his brilliant critique of the medicalization of drug problems, but brought little understanding of the flood of addiction in the modern world and how it might be brought under control.

Karl Polanyi, also an Austro-Hungarian Jew and a refugee from Europe, saw the world of menacing nation states from a communitarian rather than a libertarian viewpoint. He analyzed the roots of severe addiction (although he did not specifically use the word "addiction") and other psychological pitfalls in modern society in a more thorough way than Szasz. Although Polanyi's (1944) understanding of the roots of severe addiction was strong precisely where Szasz's was weak, Polanyi offered no analysis of the persecution and medicalization of drug users, which Szasz explained so brilliantly.

I have been exploring Polanyi's views for over a decade (for example, Alexander, 2008/2010, chap. 3; Alexander, 2010). In this chapter, I present my own, expanded version of Polanyi's insights on addiction, contrasting them with Szasz's. I hope to show that, whereas Szasz successfully unmasked a false truth about severe addiction, Polanyi unmasked one that was at least as large, and, like Szasz, advanced our critical understanding of drug use and severe addiction in an indispensable way.

Szasz and Polanyi were miles apart, philosophically and politically. Szasz abhorred European fascism as a persecuted Jew from a rich, capitalist family; Polanyi abhorred it as a persecuted Jew from a middle class family and as a passionate socialist. Szasz advocated a libertarian, atheistic, capitalist philosophy (see Szasz, 1973/1984, 2002), whereas Polanyi espoused a communitarian view with a religious base (Polanyi, 1935, 1944). Szasz focused his attention on the human need for freedom; Polanyi focussed his attention on the human need for belonging

113

and meaning. Each scholar gave voice to one of the great cries of resistance to the ugly fascism of the twentieth century—which many people fear is reemerging in the twenty-first.

Perhaps Szasz, as an impassioned libertarian, could never have been reconciled himself with Polanyi's communitarian thinking. However, I believe that reflective Szaszians in the twenty-first century can use Polanyi's insights to supplement Szasz's brilliant but incomplete analysis of severe addiction and what might be done about it. After all, the Cold War is over!

A Global, Historical View of Severe Addiction

Figure 6.1 represents a global, historical view of severe addiction within a feedback loop or "vicious cycle." In the center of the loop is an image of Karl Polanyi, because I have based this figure on Polanyi's thinking in conjunction with the evidence of historians, anthropologists, and clinicians (Alexander, 2008/2010).

Two caveats: First, the global-historical view of severe addiction is intended to explain the *societal* causes of the rising tide of severe addiction in a 500-year period that historians known as "the modern era." The global-historical view also deepens the understanding of the countless, unique individual histories of addiction and recovery.

Second, the historical view of severe addiction is not exclusively, or even primarily, about drug use. People use psychoactive drugs for diverse reasons, many of which have nothing to do with addiction. The historical perspective is about *severe addiction* to drugs or anything else.

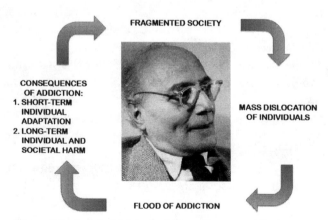

Figure 6.1. A global-historical view of severe addiction.

Fragmentation

From the time of Christopher Columbus onward, large-scale colonization by Western powers fragmented defenseless societies around the globe by conquest, disease, enslavement, economic exploitation, religious domination, and devastation of local ecosystems. This is the colonial history of the Americas, Africa, Asia, and the Middle East (Hobsbawm, 1989, chap. 3; Wright, 2004; Mann, 2011).

As the colonizing European powers conquered the globe, they also crushed defenseless subcultures *within their own countries*, although with somewhat more restraint. The demands of the agricultural and industrial revolutions and the needs of the colonial expeditions overran and crushed stable peasant villages, commons, and ethnic subcultures throughout Europe (Polanyi, 1944; El Saffar, 1994, pp. 62–68; Bollier, 2014).

The fragmentation of world society that began in the early modern era has continued to escalate right into the twenty-first century, amidst the globalization of free-market capitalism, neoliberalism, consumerism, corporate culture, enterprise culture, high-tech surveillance, ecological devastation, development, restructuring, and austerity, relentlessly increasing efficiency in manufacturing and agribusiness, unending financial crises, and neo-colonial wars (Chossudovsky, 2003; Dufour, 2003; Berardi, 2009; Harvey, 2011, pp. 66, 176; Hickinbottom-Brawn, 2013; Snowden, 2014; McWilliams, 2015, Nikiforuk, 2015; Levitin, 2015).

Global fragmentation seems inescapable because it is a side effect of an economic, political, and technological revolution that has produced enormous increases in industrial productivity and technical advancement for the human species, and has enabled the earth to support a world civilization of seven billion people. However, this brave new world is in deep, and possibly terminal trouble, in large part because of the unforeseen consequences of this fragmentation, which include dislocation and addiction.

Where Szasz's libertarian line of thought emphasized the damaging effects of national governments and large institutions on individuals, the global historical view puts the first emphasis on the damaging effects of national governments and large institutions on local societies and the *subsequent* damage to individuals who are dislocated from their social matrix. Where Szasz emphasized the damaging effects of religious inquisitions, scientific medicine, and institutional psychiatry,

Polanyi emphasized the damaging effects of colonization by European nations and the corporate institutions of the unregulated free market.

Dislocation

Following Polanyi (1944), I use the word "dislocation" to describe the *individual, psychological devastation* that follows from the fragmentation of local societies, villages, tribal groups, and clans. Dislocation refers to a form of individual malaise that can be described on many levels. In social terms it is the absence of sustaining interactions between individuals and their families and/or local societies, religions, traditions, and natural environments. In psychological terms, it is the absence of a sense of belonging, identity, meaning, and purpose, and the anxiety and depression that result. In existential terms it is the anxiety of alienation or of deep loss, the dread of "nothingness" or "non-being", or a terrifying intuition that "God is dead." In spiritual terms it can be called poverty of the spirit or a loss of faith.

Mass dislocation has tangible *benefits* for economic growth and geopolitical power. It frees individuals to perform competitively and efficiently, unimpeded by love of nature, needs for meaning or identity, or sentimental ties (Polanyi, 1944). In classical economics, this severe economic rationality is said to make the law of supply and demand function, and thus to "clear the markets" each day. Nations that have embraced the global market system in recent decades, such as China and the other BRIC nations, have rapidly become geopolitical superpowers.

Dislocation has genuine hedonistic advantages for modern individuals as well for economies. It can provide an ideal space for personal initiative, individual creativity, and self-actualization, for a time. However, prolonged, severe dislocation has a high price, because it eventually leaves people with an empty and dismal life (Polanyi, 1944; Barrett, 1962; Frankl, 1963; Erikson, 1968; Berry, 2009, pp. 35–48; Tolman, 2013; Klein, 2014, pp. 158–160; Verhaeghe, 2014).

Decrying societal fragmentation as the source of individual dislocation is more than a nostalgic lament of socialists, social workers, existentialists, historians, theologians, romantic poets, and gurus. A specific linkage between societal fragmentation and individual dislocation has been documented by scientists and investigative journalists for every stage of life, beginning before birth.

For example, severe stress endured by pregnant women in a fragmented society can render their children socially fearful years later and, hence, dislocated. Some of the brain mechanisms underlying this causal relationship have been worked out (Maté, 2008, 2015).

Lack of welcoming and reciprocal attachments to a mother, other significant adults, and age-mates—whether ultimately due to fragmentation of society or any other reason—have been demonstrated to drastically undermine a developing child's social and emotional well-being later in life (Erikson, 1963, 1968; Bowlby, 1969; Blum, 2002, chaps. 6, 7, 10).

Lack of stable housing in volatile real estate markets dominated by speculators can make integrated family and neighborhood life difficult or impossible for adults raising children. I am witnessing this first hand among my own young friends and relatives who are being dislocated by today's insanely inflated and volatile real estate market in Vancouver (see also Surowiecki, 2014; Tencer, 2015).

Work in a dehumanizing factory system, including Foxconn, where my cell phone was probably made, can leave workers so empty of meaning that suicide becomes epidemic. The nets that Foxconn has erected to save the lives of employees who leap from the factory windows are world famous (Tharoor, 2014).

Existence in a hypocritical, corrupt political system run by politicians who shamelessly serve mega-corporations and military bureaucracies leads to profound apathy in adults (Wolin, 2008; Risen, 2014). Such societies provide opportunities for demagogues who offer illusory recognition and companionship to "the ordinary guy" on an industrial scale (Towhey & Schneller, 2015).

Lack of family and neighborhood support can leave elderly people in a state of incapacitating despair (McLaren, 2014).

Severe, prolonged dislocation is unbearable. It precipitates anguish, suicide, depression, disorientation, domestic violence, and political extremism (Durkheim, 1897/1951; Polanyi, 1944; Barrett, 1962; Chandler et al., 2003; Berardi, 2009; Deraniyagala, 2013; White, 2014). Because it is unbearable, dislocation has been imposed as a dreaded punishment from ancient times to the present—banishment, solitary confinement, exile, ostracism, ex-communication. Dislocation, in the form of prolonged, radical social isolation, remains an essential component of today's terrifyingly scientific technology of torture (Klein, 2007, chap. 1; Democracy Now, 2014).

Dislocation is hard to define concisely. This is because it needs to be understood on social, psychological, existential, and spiritual levels at the same time. Moreover, it would be wrong to say that the opposite of dislocation is "normalcy" because in today's fragmented world, disloca-tion is closer to the norm. It would be simplistic to say that dislocation can be overcome by eliminating income inequality or overcoming racial prejudice and homophobia. The problem runs far deeper.

It is even harder to define what it is like *not* to be dislocated. I use the term "psychosocial integration" for the opposite of dislocation. This bit of jargon originally comes from Erik Erikson (1968). The most concise summary of Erikson's explanation of psychosocial integration that I can offer is that it is a state of balance in a well-functioning society that enables most people to be confident that they belong, yet still feel free.

Whereas Szasz eloquently described distress coming from overbear-ing governments and other large social institutions, he never, to my knowledge, dwelt on the distress that arose from breaking down local social or ethnic groups. In fact, dislocation does not fit neatly into his primary concern with a tyrannical society oppressing its outsiders, because dislocation in a fragmented world affects everybody, not just outsiders. It is here that Polanyi most obviously extends Szasz' insights.

Severe Addiction: A Way of Adapting to Dislocation

Just as high levels of dislocation follow high levels of social fragmen-tation, high levels of severe addiction inevitably follow high levels of dislocation. A wealth of historical and anthropological evidence docu-ments this sequence (Alexander, 2008/2010). Clinical and biographical evidence shows *why* severe addiction tracks dislocation so closely: Severe addictions can provide dislocated people with relief and com-pensation for their bleak existence, when nothing else seems to work (Alexander, 2008/2010, chaps. 6–8; Fetting, 2016).

When severe addictions only provide partial psychosocial integra-tion, severely dislocated people who can see no other source of relief, pursue them insatiably, even if they feel terribly guilty about the people they hurt in the process, or the other harm they do.

To say that severe addiction serves a vital adaptive function for dislocated people is not to say that it is harmless, or to make light of it. Rather, it is to explain why it is so pervasive in a fragmented and dis-located society. Many people who will never be diagnosed as addicted nonetheless recognize powerful addictive tendencies in their own lives. Addiction is neither a sin nor a disease, but intrinsic to modern society, much like competitiveness, anxiety, income inequality, and wasteful consumption.

Of course severe addiction is not the kind of adaptation that most people would choose for themselves if they could find a better alternative, or that their societies would choose for them. However, it at least provides them with some meager sense of belonging, identity, meaning, and purpose (even when it is accompanied by guilt and remorse). Without their addictions, many severely dislocated people would have terrifyingly little reason to live and might fall into incapacitating anxiety, depression, or suicide.

For example, when "junkies" wake up in the morning, they at least know who they are and what they must accomplish that day. Rather than being overwhelmed by the emptiness of their existence, they keep very, very busy chasing drugs, sometimes in collaboration with their fellow users, sometimes in competition with them. At the same time, they can hold onto a tragic but exotic junkie identity, and identify themselves with William S. Burroughs, Curt Cobain, Philip Seymour Hoffman, Amy Winehouse, Robin Williams, or Rob Ford. A kind of junkie mystique dilutes the misery of their existence with the glamorous imagery of the "tragically hip" or "the coolest" (Burroughs, 1967; Pryor, 2003).

For another example, people who are addicted to horserace gambling have not found anything more important in their lives than incessantly exchanging information and hunches within a colorful subculture of characters at the track, with a mythology of famous gamblers and legendary horses of the past and an imagined future of fabulous success (Ryan, 2014a, b).

Much larger numbers of people use drugs only moderately or go to the track recreationally. They have found more effective ways of fulfilling their needs for psychosocial integration most of the time. The tragic reality, however, is that there are countless millions of people who cannot use drugs or gamble recreationally. Their needs for belonging, identity, meaning, and purpose are so great and they seize onto these recreations avariciously, and try to build a life around them. People cling to their addictions with the same iron grip that they would apply to a piece of floating junk if they were desperately flailing for survival in a stormy sea.

The global, historical view of severe addiction entails much more than merely recognizing environmental "factors" must be taken into account in understanding a person's addiction along with the neurological effects of drugs and other factors (e.g., Reinarman & Granfield, 2015). Rather it leads to the conclusion that the flood of severe addiction in the twenty-first century can never be brought under control without seriously reducing the fragmentation and dislocation. Mass dislocation is a *sufficient cause* of mass severe addiction.

This analysis of severe addiction in the twenty-first century might not have made sense to Thomas Szasz. Here is his way of describing the causes of drug addiction in 2004 as he neared the end of his career:

> Addiction to drugs is a condition that the addict brings about by his own free will, and which he can "escape" by his own free will, with or without the aid of others . . . I see him as a capable moral agent, sometimes doing and enjoying what he wants to do and annoying others in the process, and sometimes victimizing himself or others by his behavior. (2004b, p. 196)

Szasz rejected the concept that people could get addicted to pursuits that did not entail drug use, particularly food addiction, as categorically as he insisted that drug addiction was nothing more than the free choice of a moral agent. He saw very fat and very thin people as choosing to maintain a body weight that seems to them natural, according to their own free wills. Szasz believed that the most important solution to all so-called addiction problems is more resolute application of free will (Szasz, 1973/1985, chap. 8).

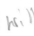

I believe that, whereas Szasz was right about the folly of medicalizing addictions of all sorts, he was wrong to put free will at the center of his analysis. Severely addicted people have not lost their will power and do not need medical treatment; they are dislocated people who have desperate needs for belonging, identity, meaning, and purpose. Addiction is the best way they have been able to find to meet these powerful needs. It can be argued legalistically that severely addicted people adopt addictive lifestyles literally "by their own free will," *but it is more useful to leave free will out of the conversation entirely,* because the *remediable* cause of addiction is not free will, but mass dislocation in a fragmented society that makes any alternative to addiction feel insufficient for growing numbers of desperate people.

Fragmenting Consequences of Severe Addiction:
The Cycle Continues

People cling to addictions because they are the best way they can find to adapt to their dislocation. However, there is an equally important, *societal* reason why the flood of severe addiction in modern society is not abating. Many of the harmful consequences of addiction exacerbate the fragmentation of modern society and, thus increase the dislocation and addiction that flows from it. The vicious cycle is completed and takes another turn.

Severe addiction exacerbates societal fragmentation in countless ways. For example, environmental and social fragmentation is steadily increased by the dictates of wealth and power addicts in the executive suites of multinational corporations that extract fossil fuels and manufacture weapons. Environmental harm and fragmentation is exacerbated by the wasteful consumption of the products of multinational manufacturing corporations by millions of their more-and-less severely addicted customers. Fragmentation is exacerbated by all the talented children who cannot be educated and socialized as productive adults because their school years have been lost to severe addictions to video games and social media. Fragmentation is exacerbated by all the adults who are lost from reflective work and citizenship because they are lost in severe addictions to money, power, drugs, sex, wealth, celebrity worship, spectator sports, fashion, pets, social networking, gambling, Internet games and so forth. Many other people are overwhelmingly involved in an endless cycle of tenuous recovery, relapse, and re-recovery. Many potentially valuable elders will not contribute their accumulated wisdom to succeeding generations because of severe addictive involvements with television, crossword puzzles, and prescription drugs.

Thus, severe addiction is not only a downstream response to societal fragmentation but also ultimately an upstream cause of it. With each new turn of the cycle, the flood of addiction rises to new heights. It is far too simple to think of severe addiction solely as a disorder that can be controlled *either* by medical therapy *or* stronger exertions of will power.

Bridging the Chasm between Szasz and Polanyi

Both Szasz and Polanyi were brilliant observers of the modern era. Both were horrified by the destruction of the human spirit that they witnessed. Polanyi focused his attention on the way that the steamroller of modernity crushed local societies that had given people a strong sense of belonging and meaning in pre-modern times. Szasz focused on the subsequent destruction of human freedom in a modern society of individuals who had already been torn from their traditional roots. He saw that not only being controlled by overt violence of enormous nation states, but also by institutionalized medical violence masked as benevolence.

Polanyi's analysis appeals more to socialists, and Szasz's to libertarians. However, they are complementary. Human beings need *both* a deep experience of belonging *and* a deep sense of freedom. This primal duality of human needs is expressed in the Judeo-Christian heritage that Szasz and Polanyi shared (see Fromm, 1941) and in great works of secular philosophy and science (Darwin, 1871/1981, chaps. 3–5; Wilson, 2012). *Both* of these fundamental needs have been ignored by many institutions of the modern world, and the human spirit has been mortified in the process.

Is it possible to conceive of a world society in the twenty-first century and beyond that neither deprives people of their basic needs for belonging nor abrogates their freedom? Of course achieving such a society goes far beyond the training of today's specialists in the field of addiction. However, both Szasz and Polanyi recognized that psychological problems, including severe addiction and its treatment, are not isolated issues whose solution can be delegated to narrow specialists and experts. They can only be fully understood in the larger context of the modern world.

Although enabling people to find a secure, meaningful place in modern society, while still feeling free, requires a delicate and complex balancing act, anthropologists have shown how this balance has been achieved in pre-modern communities and tribal groups everywhere on the planet. The balance can and must be achieved in the modern world, if human society is to complete its half-finished progression from scruffy, aggressive primate troupes to a truly compassionate, intellectual, scientific, and spiritual civilization. Finishing this progression may be necessary for the sheer survival of the species as well as its comfort. However, simply ending the War on Drugs, Institutional Psychiatry, and the Therapeutic State is not enough to get us there.

Ending Both the War on Drugs and the Flood of Addiction

The failures of the War on Drugs, Institutional Psychiatry, and the Therapeutic State to bring the addiction problem under control have been exposed again and again since Szasz's time. Their once impregnable credibility wears thin when exposed to the rough surface of reality. We can anticipate eventually looking back on the War on Drugs, Institutional Psychiatry and The Therapeutic State as nightmares receding into the past, like earlier witch-hunts and inquisitions.

But what will follow the recession of the War on Drugs, Institutional Psychiatry, and the Therapeutic State? I believe that the vision of the future that Szasz idealized in the final chapter of *Ceremonial Chemistry* is too simple. He hoped to simply move control over drugs:

> away from the [War on Drugs and the Therapeutic State] and give it to the oppressed as individuals, for each to do with as he pleases . . . as exemplified by Mill, von Mises, the free-market economists, and their libertarian followers. Revealingly, they dream of people so self-governing that their need for and tolerance of rulers is minimal or nil. (Szasz, 1973/1985, p. 177)

In the same chapter, Szasz made it clear that his libertarian dream is not limited to drugs, but applies to all human activities. He dreams of a society in which "the individual [is] treated as completely free" (Szasz, 1973/1985, p. 176).

But Szasz's libertarian vision ignores Polanyi's insights. People need belonging, identity, meaning, and purpose that they gain from membership in social groups. Social groups inevitably have rules and traditions of all sorts, often including controls over the use of psycho-active drugs. Although people need freedom, *complete* freedom soon becomes unbearable (Fromm, 1941)—as does complete domination. There is no good reason to try to force complete freedom on ourselves because the greatest achievements of human evolutionary history and of modern civilization have arisen within social organizations that limit individual freedom to a substantial extent (Darwin, 1871/1981, chaps. 3–5; Wilson, 2012). This evolutionary and historical trade-off of some potential freedom for social belonging has not only made human beings innately social, it has also made us spectacularly successful on earth.

The tragedy of twentieth-century political ideology was that it pitted people who are passionately concerned with freedom against people who are passionately concerned with belonging, rather than uniting them in the shared task of restructuring the modern world so that that is fit for habitation by human beings, in all their complexity.

The society that will solve the problem of addiction must nourish both human freedom and a deep sense of belonging. This is no easy task. Ultimately, it will require mega-scale social change. Although this kind of change must begin at the local level, it must ultimately be realized at the national and international levels as well. It will include policy innovations that are now impossible to predict.

Although it is possible that mega-scale social change may not be accomplished successfully, there is no avoiding it, because it is already underway. No matter what people concerned about addiction do, the world will continue to change in massive and presently unpredictable ways. The magnitude of the changes is already visible in the technical revolution that pervades modern life for most of us, the changing weather patterns of the planet, and the administrative changes that are envisioned in the Paris Climate Agreement of 2015 (for example, Davenport, 2015).

The essential understanding that arises from combining the insights of Szasz and Polanyi is that, if it is to have a good outcome, the process of change must take psychological realities like addiction into account, as well as the more obvious threats of ecological, political, and economic disaster. As sustainability expert Ed Ayers has pointed out: "Building a liveable world *isn't* rocket science; it's far more complex than that." (Quoted by Klein, 2014, p. 280).

The great religious and scientific thinker, Thomas Berry, has convinced me, a lifelong atheist, that the spiritual components of this transformation are as essential as the conceptual and scientific ones. As Berry put it:

> What is most needed in addition to the new technologies integrating our human needs with solar energy and the organic functioning of planetary life systems is a *deep cultural therapy* that will identify the sources of our pathology and provide a way of returning to the jubilant life expression that should characterize any human mode of being. (Berry, 2009, p. 138, emphasis added)

We cannot fully predict or plan our future. However, we can work toward it nonetheless. This work is already underway within the countless social activist, environmentalist, spiritual and social recovery groups that are each seeking to interrupt the vicious cycle in its own way (Hawken, 2007; Wilson, 2015). These groups are found around the world. The eventual fusion of this enormous pool of human energy can yield a new, more coherent civilization *that can provide a sustainable habitat for free, but psychosocially integrated human beings who will seldom be drawn into severe addictions*, as well as providing an environment in which people who have become addicted are likely to recover.

Within this vision of the future, the distinction between the problem of addiction and other, interrelated problems of modernity fades away. The task of major social change can be undertaken with hope and faith, even in the absence of a definite blueprint for the outcome, because success is possible. Does the late modern world offer a more realistic source of hope than this?

I have no plan to squeeze a detailed utopian roadmap into the ending of this chapter. I think that the future of civilization, if there is one, will be the consequence of a long period of struggle and evolution and that its final outcome is largely unpredictable. I can only contemplate a small portion of this drama, which surrounds the problem of addiction, in this chapter. I have tried to show that those who engage in this process need to take account of the brilliant insights of both Thomas Szasz and Karl Polanyi, besides many other great thinkers. Szasz and Polanyi each highlighted one of the essential needs of the human spirit. Although the two together cannot show us specifically where we are going, they can help us to see more clearly some of what must be achieved in order to get there.

Postscript #1: A Legend

I met Thomas Szasz when we both attended a conference sponsored by the Confederacy of Treaty 6 First Nations in Northern Alberta, Canada, about twenty years ago. A few other colleagues from the field of addiction also gave invited speeches, but the large audiences for the speeches were almost entirely native Indians. The talks were well-received, but the native people had ideas of their own and invited us to post-speech discussion sessions at which they voiced their concerns and critiques. The atmosphere of the conference was intense but polite, and it ended on a very good note, following an amazing concluding speech by Jeffrey A. Schaler.

One of the highlights of the conference for me was a relatively small dinner that Thomas Szasz and I both attended. It was presided over by a chief who told us a number of Cree legends, mostly unrelated to the topic of addiction. I was enthralled, but I wondered how the legends had gone over with Thomas Szasz, a champion of scientific rigor and a man who grew up in a part of the world very far removed from Northern Alberta. I asked Tom cautiously what he thought. To my surprise he replied with great enthusiasm: "It was one of the most fascinating evenings of my life!" So I feel safe in adding a native legend to my argument in this chapter, since I believe it might have made sense to Thomas Szasz.

The legend was first told to me by a native grandmother who was also a drug counselor for her reserve. The legend is that drug counselors of her tribe in northern Canada sit watchfully by the side of a raging northern mountain river. When they see somebody being swept away in the raging white foam of addiction they jump in to rescue them.

They know how to swim through the rapids to the drowning swimmer because their elders have told them where the rocks are hidden. Using all their strength, they eventually reach the addicted person and drag him or her through the torrent to the shore and with their last ounce of strength heave him or her up on the bank.

Sometimes the effort is wasted. The addicted person slips off the riverbank and is lost again in the foam. But sometimes he or she stands up and walks from the river into the forest, rejoining the people and the land.

When someone is saved, the storyteller told me, counselors swell with pride. They feel that they are warriors! They would feel that they are making a great contribution to their people except . . .

> Except, she said, that *some son-of-a-bitch upstream* is throwing more and more people into the water all the time! The counselors eventually realize that they are not winning but losing, for all their heroic efforts, but they persist anyway.

I believe that we who care about addiction must continue the heroic rescue work, but I also believe that the even more essential task is getting rid of "the-son of-a-bitch upstream," that is, the vicious cycle that is described by the global, historical view of severe addiction.

Postscript #2: Institutional Indignation Drones on in the Background

Thomas Szasz has embarrassed the huge multiprofessional/governmental complex that he called "Institutional Psychiatry" and the "Therapeutic State" by exposing the hypocrisy of those within it who represent themselves as "pure scientists" whose completely objective research is uninfluenced by the mammoth power of culture and politics. They look even sillier when they profess that they act solely in the interests of their patients or clients, denying how much they also strive for material rewards and professional status. Only *one* punishment could be severe enough for Szasz's repeated, scathing, public exposure of this hypocrisy . . . but he has escaped it!

Szasz has avoided being burned at the stake by arranging to die at home. However, those who still support the hypocrisy of the Therapeutic State can immolate him in their hearts and by caricaturing him in professional discourse and classrooms forever. They will not feel that they are being cruel in administering this eternal punishment of his heresy. Moreover, I can imagine that he could only be amused to learn that he is being made a posthumous victim at virtual *autos-de-fé* in the twenty-first century.

So let Institutional Psychiatry burn him in perpetuity! Ultimately, however, we will relearn that the tools of the Inquisition can only destroy the heretics, but never the heresy. Rather, Inquisitions keep the heresy alive by dramatizing it symbolically in the consuming flames. Is this not why Inquisitions fail in the end? In burning and reburning Szasz, his heresy of exposing pseudoscience and pseudosaintliness will be kept alive!

Ultimately, thanks to Thomas Szasz and others who have dared to tell the truth, those who have served the psychiatric and psychological professions may eventually see clearly enough to assume the truly useful public role that is open to us once we overcome our compulsive medicalizing.

References

Ahmed, S. H., Lenoir, M., & Guillem, K. (2013). Neurobiology of addiction versus drug use driven by lack of choice. *Current Opinion in Neurobiology, 23*, 581–587.

Alexander, B. K. (2008/2010). *The globalization of addiction: A study in poverty of the spirit*. Oxford: Oxford University Press.

Alexander, B. K. (2010). Addiction as seen from the perspective of Karl Polanyi. Retrieved December 10, 2015, from www .brucekalexander.com/articles-speeches/dislocation-theory-addiction /215-addictionseenfromkarlpolanyi

Alexander, B. K. (2014). The rise and fall of the official view of addiction. Retrieved July 26, 2015, from http://www.brucekalexander.com /articles-speeches/277-rise-and-fall-of-the-official-view-of-addiction-6

Alexander, B. K. (2015). Addiction, environmental crisis, and global capitalism. Retrieved August 14, 2015 from www.brucekalexander.com/articles -speeches/283-addiction,-environmental-crisis,-and-global-capitalism

Alexander, B. K., & Schweighofer, A. R. F. (1988). Defining 'addiction'. *Canadian Psychology, 29*, 151–162.

Alexander, B. K., & Shelton, C. P. (2014). *A history of psychology in western civilization*. Cambridge: Cambridge University Press.

Berardi, F. (2009). *Precarious rhapsody: Semiocapitalism and the pathologies of the post-alpha generation*. Brooklyn, NY: Autonomedia.

Barrett, W. (1962). *Irrational man: A study in existential philosophy*. Garden City, NY: Doubleday Anchor Books.

Berry, T. (2009). *The sacred universe: Earth, spirituality, and religion in the twenty-first century*. New York: Columbia University Press.

Blum, D. (2002). *Love at Goon Park: Harry Harlow and the science of affection*. Cambridge, MA: Perseus.

Bollier, D. (2014). *Think like a commoner: A short introduction to the life of the commons*. Gabriola Island, BC: New Society Publishers.

Bowlby, J. (1969). *Attachment.* Volume I of *Attachment and loss.* New York: Basic Books.

Burroughs, W. S. (1967, July). Kicking drugs: A very personal story. *Harper's, 235,* 39–42.

Case, A., & Deaton, A. (2015). Rising morbidity and mortality in midlife among white non-Hispanic Americans in the 21st century. *PNAS (Proceedings of the National Academy of Sciences),* Retrieved November 8, 2015, from http://www.pnas.org/content/early/2015/10/29/1518393112

Chandler, M. J., Lalonde, C. E., Sokol, B. W., & Hallet, D. (2003). Personal persistence, identity development, and suicide: A study of native and non-native north American adolescents. *Monographs of the Society for the Study of Child Development, 68*(2), 1–130.

Chossudovsky, M. (2003).*The globalization of poverty: Impact of IMF and World Bank reforms.* London: Zed.

Cohen, P. (2000). *Is the addiction doctor the voodoo priest of western man?* CEDRO: Centrum voor drogssonderzoek. Retrieved December 10, 2011, from www.cedro-uva.org/lib/cohen.addiction.html

Darwin, C. (1981). *The descent of man, and selection in relation to sex.* Princeton, NJ: Princeton University Press. (Original work published 1871).

Davenport, C. (2015, December 13). A climate deal, 6 fateful years in the making. *The New York Times,* Retrieved December 14, 2015, from http://www.nytimes.com/2015/12/14/world/europe/a-climate-deal-6-fateful-years-in-the-making.html?_r=0

Democracy Now. (March 18, 2014). A sliver of light: Freed U.S. hikers on captivity in Iran & activism against solitary confinement (Amy Goodman interview). Retrieved December 12, 2015, from http://www.democracynow.org/2014/3/18/a_sliver_of_light_freed_us

Deraniyagala, S. (2013). *Wave: A memoir* (pp. 55–59). Toronto: McClelland & Stewart.

Dufour, D.-R. (2003). *L'art de réduire les têtes; Sur la nouvelle servitude de l'homme libéré à l'ere du capitalisme total.* Paris: Édition Nöel.

Durkheim, E. 1951. *Suicide: A study in sociology* (J.A. Spaulding & G. Simpson, Trans.). Glencoe, IL: Free Press (original work published 1897).

El Saffar, R. A. (1994). *Rapture encaged: The suppression of the Feminine in western culture.* New York: Routledge.

Erikson, E. H. (1963). *Childhood and society* (2nd ed.). New York: Norton.

Erikson, E. H. (1968). *Identity, youth and crisis.* New York: Norton.

Fetting, M. (2016). *Perspectives on substance use, disorders, and addiction: With clinical cases* (2nd ed.). London: Sage.

Frances, A. (2013). *Saving normal: An insider's revolt against out-of-control psychiatric diagnosis, DSM-5, big pharma, and the medicalization of ordinary life.* New York: William Morrow (HarperCollins).

Google Books. (undated). Google books ngram viewer. Retrieved February 1, 2016, from https://books.google.com/ngrams/info

Frankl, V. E. (1963). *Man's search for meaning: An introduction to logotherapy.* New York: Pocket Books.

Fromm, E. (1941). *Escape from freedom.* New York: Holt, Rinehart, and Winston

Hall, W., Carter, A., & Forini, C. (2015). The brain disease model of addiction: Is it supported by the evidence and has it delivered on its promises? *The Lancet: Psychiatry, 2,* 105–110.

Hari, J. (2015). *Chasing the scream: The first and last days of the war on drugs.* London: Bloomsbury.

Hart, C. (2013). *High price: A neuroscientist's voyage of self-discovery that challenges everything you know about drugs and society.* New York: HarperCollins.

Harvey, D. (2011). *The enigma of capital and the crises of capitalism.* London: Profile Books.

Hawken, P. (2007). *Blessed unrest: How the largest social movement in the world came into being.* New York: Viking.

Hickinbottom-Brawn, S. (2013). Brand "you": The emergence of social anxiety disorder in the age of enterprise. *Theory and Psychology, 23.* Retrieved October 31, 2015, from http://tap.sagepub.com/content/23/6/732

Hobsbawm, E. J. (1989). *The age of empire: 1875–1914.* New York: Random House (Vintage).

Klein, N. (2007). *The shock doctrine: The rise of disaster capitalism.* Toronto, ON: Knopf.

Klein, N. (2014). *This changes everything: Capitalism vs. the climate.* Toronto, ON: Knopf, Canada.

Levitin, D. J. (2015). Why the modern world is bad for your brain. *The Guardian (The Observer),* Retrieved January 18, 2015, from http://www.theguardian.com/science/2015/jan/18/modern-world-bad-for-brain-daniel-j-levitin-organized-mind-information-overload

Levy, N. (2013). Addiction is not a brain disease (and it matters). *Frontiers in Psychiatry, 4*(article 24), 1–6.

Mann, C. C. (2011). *1493: Uncovering the new world Columbus created.* New York: Vintage Books.

Maté, G. (2008). *In the realm of hungry ghosts: Close encounters with addiction* (pp. 205–207). Toronto, ON: Knopf.

Maté, G. (2015). Toxic cultures | bioneers. Youtube. Retrieved March 29, 2015, from https://youtu.be/erZhTPkOLb

McLaren, L. (2014, March 17). All the lonely old people. *Maclean's, 127*(10), 36.

McWilliams, J. (2015, Spring). Inside big ag: On the dilemma of the meat. *Virginian Quarterly Review.* Retrieved July 29, 2015, from www.vqronline.org/nonfiction-criticism/2015/04/inside-big-ag-dilemma-meat-industry

Munro, D. (2015). Inside the $35 billion addiction treatment industry. *Forbes.* Retrieved December 4, 2015, from http://www.forbes.com/sites/danmunro/2015/04/27/inside-the-35-billion-addiction-treatment-industry/

Nature editorial. (2014, February 5). Animal farm: Europe's policy-makers must not buy animal-rights activists' arguments that addiction is a social, rather than a medical, problem. *Nature, 506*(7486). Retrieved April 1, 2014, from www.nature.com/news/animal-farm-1.14660

Nikiforuk. (2015, January 10). Fracking industry shakes up Northern BC with 231 tremors. *The Tyee*. Retrieved January 17, from http://thetyee.ca /News/2015/01/10/Fracking_Industry_Shakes_Up_Northern_BC/

Oxford English Dictionary. (2010). Oxford: Oxford University Press.

Pearson, H. (2004, 22 July) Science and the war on drugs: A hard habit to break. *Nature, 430*, 394–395.

Peele, S. (1989). *The diseasing of America: Addiction treatment out of control*. Lexington, MA: Lexington Books.

Pickard, H. (2012, April 18). The purpose in chronic addiction. *AJOB Neuroscience, 3*(2), 40–49. Retrieved August 15, 2015, from www.ncbi.nlm. nih.gov/pmc/articles/PMC3378040/

Polanyi, K. (1935). The essence of fascism. In J. Lewis, K. Polanyi, & D. K. Kitchin, (Eds.), *Christianity and the social revolution* (pp. 359–394). London: Victor Gollancz.

Polanyi, K. (1944). *The great transformation: The political and economic origins of our times*. Boston, MA: Beacon.

Pryor, W. (2003). *The survival of the coolest: An addiction memoir*. Bath: Clear Press.

Reinarman, C., & Granfield, R. (2015). Addiction is not just a brain disease: Critical studies of addiction. In R. Granfield & C. Reinarman (Eds.), *Expanding addiction: Critical essays* (pp. 1–21). New York: Taylor & Francis (Routledge).

Risen, J. (2014). *Pay any price: Greed, power, and endless war*. New York: Houghton, Mifflin, Harcourt.

Roth, C. (1964). *The Spanish inquisition*. New York: Oxford University Press. (Original work published 1937).

Ryan, D. (2014a, April 26). Hastings Park gallops on: The glory days are gone but Vancouver's racetrack still has its own unique community. *The Vancouver Sun*, B11–B12.

Ryan, D. (2014b, April 26). Living the life: The mystical beauty of horses and family of racetrack personalities captivate Vancouver author Kevin Chong. *The Vancouver Sun*, B12.

Satel, S., & Lilienfeld, S. C. (2013). *Brainwashed: The seductive appeal of mindless neuroscience*. New York: Basic Books.

Schaler, J. A. (2000). *Addiction is a choice*. Chicago, IL: Open Court.

Seelye, K. Q. (2015, October 30). In heroin crisis, white families seek gentler War on Drugs. *The New York Times*. Retrieved November 24, 2015, from http://www.nytimes.com/2015/10/31/us/heroin-war-on-drugs-parents. html?_r=0W

Snowden, E. (2014, June 7). How the national security state kills a free society. Reader supported news. Retrieved June 7, 2014, from: http://readersup-portednews.org/opinion2/277-75/24094-how-the-national-security-state-kills-a-free-society

Surowiecki, J. (2014, June 26). Real estate goes global. *The New Yorker*. Retrieved June 4, 2014, from www.newyorker.com/talk/financial/2014 /05/26/140526ta_talk_surowiecki

Sussman, S., Lisha, N., & Griffiths, M. (2010). Prevalence of the addictions: A problem of the majority or the minority? US National Library of Medicine, NCBI. Retrieved November 22, 2015, from www.ncbi.nlm.nih.gov/pmc /articles/PMC3134413/

Szasz, T. S. (1970). *The manufacture of madness: A comparative study of the inquisition and the mental health movement.* New York: Dell (Delta).

Szasz, T. S. (1973/1985). *Ceremonial chemistry: The ritual persecution of drugs, addicts, and pushers* (Rev. Ed.). Holmes Beach, FL: Learning Publications (original publication 1973).

Szasz, T. S. (2002, June). *Hayek and psychiatry. Liberty, 16,* 19–20 and 24.

Szasz, T. S. (2004a). An autobiographical sketch. In J. A. Schaler (Ed.), *Szasz under fire: The psychiatric abolitionist faces his critics* (pp. 1–28). Chicago: Open Court.

Szasz, T. S. (2004b). Reply to Peele. In J. A.Schaler (Ed.), *Szasz under fire: The psychiatric abolitionist faces his critics* (pp. 196–197). Chicago: Open Court.

Tencer. (2015, November 3). 5 signs Canada's housing markets are out of control. *Huffington Post.* Retrieved November 4, 2015, from http://www .huffingtonpost.ca/2015/11/03/canada-housing-market_n_8461888 .html?utm_hp_ref=canada-business

Tharoor. (2014, November 12). The haunting poetry of a Chinese factory worker who committed suicide. *The Washington Post.* Retrieved November 16, 2014, from http://www.washingtonpost.com/blogs/worldviews /wp/2014/11/12/the-haunting-poetry-of-a-chinese-factory-worker-who -committed-suicide/

Tolman, C. W. (2013). Sumus ergo sum: The psychology of self and how Descartes got it wrong. In W. E. Smythe (Ed.), *Toward a psychology of persons* (pp. 3–24). New York: Psychology Press.

Towhey, M., & Schneller, J. (2015). *Mayor Rob Ford: Uncontrollable.* New York: Skyhorse.

Verhaeghe, P. (2014, October 3–9). Neoliberal economy brings out worst in us. *The Guardian Weekly,* 18.

White, P. (2014, December 6). Solitary: A death sentence. *The Globe and Mail,* F1-F9.

Wilson, E. O. (2012). *The social conquest of earth.* New York: Liveright (Norton).

Wilson, G. (2015). The globalization of addiction and responses that move toward recovery. Retrieved December 31, 2015, from www.brucekalexander .com

Wolin, S. S. (2008). *Democracy incorporated: Managed democracy and the specter of inverted totalitarianism.* Princeton, NJ: Princeton University Press.

Wright, J. (2004). *God's soldiers: Adventure, politics, intrigue, and power—A history of the Jesuits.* New York: Doubleday.

7

Szaszian Reflections on Cults

Jeffrey A. Schaler

Doublethink means the power of holding two contradictory beliefs in one's mind simultaneously, and accepting both of them . . . These contradictions are not accidental, nor do they result from ordinary hypocrisy: they are deliberate exercises in doublethink. For it is only by reconciling contradictions that power can be retained indefinitely . . . If human equality is to be forever averted—if the High, as we have called them, are to keep their places permanently—then the prevailing mental condition must be controlled insanity. (Orwell, 1981)

Freedom and Responsibility

Many people believe that cults are created and led by power-hungry, hypnotic, charismatic leaders, and that membership in a cult consists of adherents who are "brainwashed," and seduced, as well as coerced into maintaining involvement and allegiance to the group and its leader. This refers to the "conventional wisdom" about cults. It is a misunderstanding based on the idea that human behavior can be automatic, unconscious, like that of a machine, a thing.

Behavior, as Thomas Szasz was fond of saying repeatedly has *reasons*. Things, that is, inanimate objects, machines, for example, are *caused*. Human behavior, as described elsewhere by Thomas Szasz and others, for example, by Professor of Philosophy Emeritus Herbert Fingarette (personal communication), is the expression of human values or moral agency, a choice. When we hold a person responsible for his behaviors, we recognize the role of intent, choice made by a moral agent. The more freedom to choose, the more responsibility we believe is necessary. If there was a core principle to all of Szasz's writings and life work it was, I believe, that of moral agency and its relation to responsibility, and responsibility in turn to liberty or freedom.

Freedom and responsibility are positively correlated. The more freedom a person has, the more responsible he is for his behavior.

The less freedom a person has, the less responsible he is. Think of a person in prison. He is deprived of his freedom. He is also deprived of responsibility for room and board. He does not have to work to collect money to pay for expenses necessary for his survival. This is why some people do not mind being in prison. I have worked with people in psychotherapy holding that view.

The myth used here is that freedom is negatively correlated with responsibility. In the Orwellian world of Nineteen Eighty-Four, doublethink, that is, contradiction, is used to convince people they can be free by abdicating responsibility. Or that they can be responsible by abdicating freedom. A similar situation to prison is found in a cult, in varying degrees. A person abdicates freedom by agreeing not to disagree with the status quo of the group. As a result, responsibility for life is no longer an individual issue. Since the individual, in his mind, becomes confluent with the group, the group shares responsibility. The difference is that in a cult, the cell door is unlocked, and the metaphorical inmate can walk out any time he so chooses.

Again, Szasz has asserted that behavior has reasons. In my opinion this cannot be overstated when discussing and applying Szasz's ideas. Things are caused. There are reasons for all behaviors and because people constitute a heterogeneous society, the reasons for behaviors vary tremendously. When people assert that aberrant behavior is caused, they are referring to the person as a thing. For example, applied to drug consuming behavior, people use drugs in different ways, for different reasons, with different results. Everyone is different. A myth regarding drug users is that the population of drug users is homogeneous. If we regard the population as homogeneous, we must do the same thing to everyone in order to help them, if they want help. When we say that something or someone caused someone to do such and such, we mean that what he does, for example joining a group called a cult, is not a choice, his involvement was caused, usually by some powerful other, who affected his brain in some as of yet unknown way, the way that a machine causes things to happen. Even when people ran away from the collapsing twin towers on 9/11, their running-away-behavior was a choice, in the face of danger and certain death. In a "gun-to-the-head-scenario," people still choose to live or die. French philosopher Albert Camus (1913–60) posed one of the best-known existential questions, in his novel, The Myth of Sisyphus: "There is only one really serious philosophical question, and that is suicide." Szasz was fond of this and similar sayings. The philosopher William Barrett discussed the idea that man is a machine, based on a series of automatic, preplanned decisions, executed one after another, the way an automobile engine is caused, one event after another, one series of preprogrammed decisions or actions after another, in his book entitled *The Illusion of Technique* (1979). The last thing we want from a machine is for it to be spontaneous or creative. The view that man is a machine is based on a mechanistic philosophy, where every action termed behavior is reduced to chemical and electrical interactions. Man is said to be a machine, an incredibly complex machine but a machine nevertheless.

Mechanists eschew the idea that man has a soul, or an invisible field of energy, that ultimately maintains health and when weakened, allegedly is a cue to disease and sickness. I do not maintain that I agree with this philosophy and explanation for health and disease. I only offer it as a major explanation for health and illness by which much of the world abides. The bottom line is that we do not know whether chemicoelectrical interactions are the cause or product of behavior. The same is true for putative low levels of serotonin in depression, for example. Do alleged (unproven) low levels of serotonin cause depression, or is it the other way around? Just because a drug increases the amount of serotonin in the action potential, and a person may feel less depressed, by no means proves that he had low levels of serotonin which caused depression.

This philosophy or view of man may be compared to a vitalistic philosophy, the élan vital discussed by Henri Bergson; and/or to the gestalt psychology philosophy used to explain perception, where "the whole of man is greater than the sum of its parts." Something "holds" the parts together, be it context, in the eye of the beholder, whatever. In traditional Chinese medicine this metaphorical glue is referred to as "chi." In ancient Ayurvedic Indian medicine it was called "prajna." Homeopaths called it "the vital force." None of these terms, names, or labels were accurate or descriptive, though. They each referred to that something which made the whole greater than the sum of its parts. We don't know what that "something" is, and perhaps we never will. Call it mind, soul, energy, who knows. This "it," perhaps best described as "that represented by the pronoun 'I,'" in my opinion, is not only the essence of moral agency, it is the essence of what makes a person human, that constituting man as a moral agent. Once we recognize which philosophy we are operating from, the mechanistic or the vitalistic, we are obliged to explain behavior and human phenomena accordingly, in ways that are consistent with that underlying Weltanschauung or "world view."

Consciousness is not something that can be adequately explained by neuroscience. People mistakenly criticized Szasz for being a mind–body Cartesian dualist. Szasz and I spoke about this frequently. It makes no sense to speak of a body-less mind, he would say. That would be a ghost or spirit, and we don't believe in ghosts. A mindless body is a dead body. The closest I can come to identifying the origin of moral agency is to call it "that represented by the pronoun 'I." For the purposes of this discussion, it seems to me this point of view is best represented by the word choice. Man chooses to do x, y, and z for reasons that are important to him. The reasons are different from person to person because no two people are identical. (This is why, in part, some people regard "social science" as a contradiction. In their opinion, one cannot *accurately* generalize or infer behavioral characteristics from one person to another because people are too different from one another.)

Brain and Mind

One other operational definition seems necessary here. Brain and mind are different. People mistakenly call the mind brain and vice versa. Brain is a thing, a literal physical organ. Brains do not act or behave, they have no moral agency. We find evidence of brain disease in a corpse during autopsy by lesions caused by disease. There is no sign of mind, of irrational behavior, excessive drinking or smoking. The effects of an activity may exist in the body.

Strictly speaking, as Szasz repeatedly said, there is no such thing as the mind. While neuroscientists are fond of talking about the neurochemistry of consciousness, no such relationship can exist without committing what Gilbert Ryle referred to as a category error or mistake. The language of physicality does not translate to the language of mind or consciousness in a meaningful or accurate way. When someone asserts that brain causes mind, or vice versa, meaning that brain causes meaningful behavior, in our case, mental illness or cult behavior, they are mistaken.

While a cult often has religious characteristics and is often bound together by contradictory religious beliefs—though contradictory beliefs do not necessarily have to exist for a group to be a cult, any more contradictory than noncult beliefs—what Orwell described as "doublethink" in his novel *1984*, and the cult is frequently something of a closed or secret society, it doesn't have to be religious. Psychiatrically speaking, members appear to have schizoaffective tendencies, a "spaced out stare," a far-away look, they often manifest what Wilhelm

Reich termed the "schizophrenic gaze" (Reich, 1945). Followers tend to use the same language and figures of speech—adjectives, adverbs, metaphors, and intonations expressed by their charismatic leaders or influential other group members, when there is no leader. They are like programmed robots, as if they are machines—but they are human beings, not things.

In early writings on Gestalt Therapy this tendency to act like the other is called introjection (Perls, 1947). It is usually viewed by outsiders and "cult deprogrammers" as an unconscious, involuntary process. Members appear to be in a trance. Followers tend to "swallow whole" or introject the language and behaviors of a celebrated leader, or someone that is admired by others in the group if there is no leader, someone usually considered superhuman. They identify by trying to be like their leader, or again, in leaderless cults like Alcoholics Anonymous (AA), like those they admire, often called "elders" in AA, or "old timers."

The purpose of this essay is to reflect on how cults function in ways that are often different from conventional wisdom, using ideas about moral agency and behavior applied to human beings as developed throughout Szasz's writings. If there is one constant that runs through all of Szasz's writings it is that human behavior is an expression of choice, the exercise of free will. Group and individual membership in the cult is conscious, voluntary, and a choice, and it cannot be otherwise. While some critics of Szasz have defined mental illness as irrational behavior, we must consider Szasz's response to such assertions: Irrational according to whom? (personal communication) In other words, one person may view another's behavior as irrational. Another person may view that same person's behavior as rational. Rational or irrational is a judgment, something subjective, not objective.

Behavior means mode of conduct, or deportment. There is no such thing as an involuntary behavior. *All* behaviors are conscious and willful. Behaviors are different from convulsion or seizures. The former are willful, the latter are neurological reflexes, autonomic expressions. The patellar-knee reflex is not a behavior. Neither is an epileptic seizure.

The Rule of Cults

Contemporary mainstay religions have many of the characteristics of cults, as do many secular groups. There are socially acceptable cults and socially unacceptable ones, just as there are socially acceptable self-reported imaginings, for example, religious claims and beliefs, and socially unacceptable ones, for example, the hallucinations reported by people diagnosed as schizophrenic. One person may claim that he is "born again," or that "Jesus Christ has entered his heart." Another may claim there are alien beings from distant galaxies masquerading as pink elephants walking upside down on the ceiling. Both are hallucinations or self-reported imaginings. The religious hallucination is often considered socially acceptable, appropriate as part of religious belief (as long as one does not go too public discussing them). The hallucination or claim by someone *labeled* as schizophrenic is considered socially unacceptable. People tend to call socially unacceptable groups "cults." Socially acceptable groups are obviously viewed favorably. Mistaking the metaphor for something literal is what Szasz called "literalizing the metaphor." Sick behavior does not refer to disease, it refers to behavior judged bad. A sick joke cannot be treated with antibiotics. Spring fever is not the indication of infection.

The main way groups are held together in cults is through the prohibition placed on the expression of disagreement with the unifying ideology and identity. The rule of cults, "thou shalt not disagree" is most characteristic of all cults. Break the rule, and you break the spell. It is also a rule among socially acceptable groups. As we shall see, Thomas Szasz broke the rule regarding the cult of institutional psychiatry. (Like Szasz, I differentiate between institutional psychiatry and consensual or contractual psychiatry. In the former, a psychiatrist claiming to be an agent of the patient, is really the agent of the state or a third party, parents, for example. In the latter, there is no third party. The psychiatrist is an agent of the patient, and can be fired at any time by the patient.)

What Is a Cult?

A group is here defined as a cult when its members place a high value on sharing a unitary identity and have no tolerance for an opposing point of view. Disagreement is punished. "Cult" is generally considered a derogatory term, used to criticize the way two or more people gather together and share beliefs about themselves and the world, through an exchange of ideas, philosophy, rituals, tenets to guide one's daily life, and so on, often at the expense of individual autonomy. The cult occupies a place in a member's life similar to that of a socially acceptable religion. This is usually accomplished through the use of some discipline to strengthen beliefs and allegiance to a group (See the chapters "Busting the Disease-Model Cult" and "Addiction Treatment and the First Amendment," in Schaler, 2000). As Henry Zvi Lothane has pointed out elsewhere, it takes two persons to make a psychiatric diagnosis and one person to have a disease like cancer or heart disease. This distinction is important. For psychiatric diagnosis-making, as well as cult "group-think" is a function of group formation and social interaction, as well as labeling. Labeling, as sociologists have long known to be true, is a powerful way of stigmatizing outsiders and those who fall out of favor with the doublethink or group think of the cult. Cult-like behavior is a normal manifestation of humans interacting in groups. It has its dangers, which ought to be watched, and cannot be accurately condemned out of hand as wholly bad. My own view of cults is that they are bad. Expressing difference of opinion is a virtue, in my opinion. Punishing people for their different point of view is a vice.

Cults can also be political, psychological, psychotherapeutic, medical, atheistic, you name it—most any group of people can become a cult—as long as there is emphasis on a singular identity and enforcement of group think, with the rule, "thou shalt not disagree." Cults and sects are different, though some people equate the two. A religious sect is not necessarily viewed by others in a derogatory fashion. "Cult" implies something considered bad if not dangerous. A Jewish cult may very well view the Anglo-American cult of Christianity as a new manifestation of an old social problem, as long as the larger, and older group members express stigmatizing power against Jews.

Cargo Cult Science

If you are doing an experiment, you should report everything that might make it invalid, not just those things that support your hypothesis or theory, or not only those things that you think are right about it, as Richard Feynman explained (1974, http://calteches.library.caltech.edu/51/2/CargoCult.htm). If you want to build a safe that is impossible to break into, one should try to break into it, to test the security, the resistance to break in. Computer firewalls that are allegedly free from hackers should be tested by hiring experts to see if they can break into the computer.

Feynman discussed Pacific south sea islanders who tried to replicate American and other Westerner bases used during World War II with wood and coconuts in place of workable machines and instruments, in order to facilitate what they believed would be the return of goods and supplies they acquired and benefited from during occupation. By building something that looked very similar to the actual air and troop bases, they thought valued goods and supplies would reappear. They believed the cargo, which ought to come to them from the gods, had been diverted by Westerners and if the islanders did what the Westerners were observed to be doing, the cargo would come to them, as it rightfully should.

A similar cargo cult may be seen as existing among psychiatrists and other mental health professionals who are convinced they are diagnosing and treating physical disease in the name of psychiatric disease. Psychiatric disease looks like literal disease to those mental health professionals believing in it. Yet, the diseases don't actually exist. There is only abnormal behavior, the metaphor of disease. Psychiatrists and others who believe that metaphorical diseases are literal diseases seem to think that if they act as though they were diagnosing and treating real disease, despite the fact these were metaphorical diseases, then perhaps these mental diseases would become real diseases, and the psychiatrists would be acting as real doctors. They are literalizing the disease metaphor. In this way, institutional psychiatrists and others who believe they are diagnosing and treating a disease are similar to the south sea islanders Feynman referred to.

People believe in mental illness the way they believe in God, or the way they believe in magnetism or gravity. The belief functions as an explanation for events and activities that are difficult if not impossible to understand. People abhor a vacuum when it comes to explaining upsetting events and disturbing behaviors. Saying a person is disturbed is more comforting than saying that a person's behavior is disturbing. Showing the disease does not actually exist is tantamount to atheism. People get very upset with atheists. Similarly, people got very upset with Szasz, and get upset with people who share Szasz's thoughts concerning the meaning of behavior and disease, as well as the policies based on his discoveries.

A valid hypothesis is a falsifiable hypothesis, as Sir Karl Popper articulated. Popper maintained that if a theory is not falsifiable, it does not belong to empirical science, although it might still be meaningful and possibly true. It would possibly belong to metaphysics and shouldn't try to be scientific. We should just be clear that it is not science. Like belief in God, psychiatric diagnoses are not falsifiable. This core principle of the scientific method, falsification, is something absent in cult theories about the world and being human. After all, there is usually an unspoken taboo against falsification. Consider the similarity with Christian Science. Adherents in this religion eschew modern medicine, and believe that prayer and devotion to God heals and cures real disease. If the treatment did not work, it is allegedly due to a failure in prayer effort. In theories based on science we search for problems that render the theory false, not the other way around, that is, not for evidence supporting a theory. In antiscientific theories, falsification is forbidden. That is one of the core differences between scientific and nonscientific-based theories. I submit that the cult known as institutional psychiatry is based on the rejection of falsification.

The Cult of Psychiatry: Szasz Broke the Rule

For example, when Thomas Szasz wrote and published *The Myth of Mental Illness*, the Commissioner of the New York State Department of Mental Hygiene, Paul H. Hoch, tried to have him removed from the medical university where Szasz was a tenured professor (see http://ahrp. org/nypsi-an-early-cia-contracted-academic-institution-under-mk -naomi/). Hoch directed the chairman of the Department of Psychiatry at Upstate Medical University in Syracuse, NY, Marc Hollender, to get rid of Szasz. Szasz's falsification of psychiatry was forbidden and punished. Szasz's writings destabilized the beliefs and theories that held the world of institutional psychiatry together (Schaler, 2004). Szasz broke an unspoken rule regarding the cult of psychiatry. Thou shalt not show how mental illness does not exist. By breaking that rule he also exposed the psychiatric profession as a cult. Science always has some cult-like features.

Today, any academic who challenges the disease model theory of psychiatry, psychology, and addiction through writings, teaching, and speeches is likely to not be hired for an academic position, fired from an academic position, or refused federal funding for a research project. I know this is true because it happened to me. My contract to teach as a fulltime professor at several major universities was not renewed because I taught most every aspect of Szasz's ideas in approximately fourteen different undergraduate and graduate level courses at four different colleges and universities. The fact that students loved my classes, and that I consistently received the highest evaluations throughout each university, plus had more publications than any other member of our department faculty, was apparently irrelevant. Defamatory rumors were spread. Many colleagues of mine who are exceptionally good professors have reported similar experiences. It is considered "dangerous" to teach Szasz. While students are always excited to learn about Szasz's ideas, faculty and administrators are frequently upset. The more effective and popular the professor, the more likely he is to be harassed or fired. Aside from popularity jealousy, this is most likely to occur because

141

Szasz's ideas again undermine the theoretical bases upon which most theories of psychology and psychologically based public policy, including law, are based. On more than one occasion students of mine told me of how I was denounced by a psychology professor for teaching Szaszian perspectives on mental illness, institutional psychiatry, and related matters. "Professor Schaler is crazy," asserted more than one psychology professor. And in one forensic psychology class taught by a professor in my department, he apparently began each semester by announcing to his students that he would not address any question from students that came about as a result from attending my classes. Interestingly, the student who relayed this to me, herself a psychology major who often argued with me in class, said that she got up in one psychology class and said to her professor, "you may not agree with Dr. Schaler's point of view, however, he is not 'crazy.'" (I taught for about twenty-four years in the School of Public Affairs, Department of Justice, Law and Society at American University in Washington, DC, never in the psychology department. Psychology majors frequently attended my classes because, as they said, they wanted a different point of view. Many students subsequently dropped their psychology major as a result of taking my classes. I never once encouraged a student to drop his major. I always told my students never to *believe* anything I said in class simply because I said it, but to investigate the veracity of what I taught on their own.)

Cult Characteristics

Sometimes a charismatic leader is present in a cult, sometimes not. There is no charismatic leader in Alcoholics Anonymous (AA), for example. Yet AA is often considered a cult, and this free, spiritual self-help fellowship shares many of the characteristics of cults in general. Some psychiatrists and psychologists are very critical of cults, especially those groups they call cults that criticize institutional psychiatry, and tell people that psychiatrists are dangerous. The Church of Scientology and American and European psychiatrists have long battled one another (Louis Jolyon West, 1991). People who have been forced into AA by the state for drunk driving or driving-while-intoxicated often consider it a cult. Ideas and opinions inconsistent with the "loss of control theory of alcoholism," the cornerstone of the disease concept of alcoholism, are not only forbidden but the people expressing them are punished (Schaler, 2000). Mainstream religions often call nontraditional offshoots of their religion, offshoots that are not sanctioned by a mainstream religion, cults. Calling a group a cult is a way of stigmatizing and controlling the group and its members, as well as its ideas. Stigma here refers to a deeply discrediting attribute.

According to one expert on the sociology of religion, however, AA is like churches affiliated with the Southern Baptist Convention, in that while to outsiders, the whole movement is seen as an entity which does things within the movement, nearly everything happens at the local small-scale level. Thus, in any given Southern Baptist church, one may find one or two dominant personalities, but not in the denomination as a whole. The same may be true of AA. A religious sect is not necessarily viewed by others in a derogatory fashion. "Cult" usually implies something dangerous (Galanter, 1989; Singer & Lalich, 1995).

My own view of AA as a religious activity and/or cult is that this is not necessarily a problem, as long as people choose to go into the program and choose to stay. Most all religions are based on myth. AA becomes a serious problem when the state orders citizens into the program. Then the state violates the establishment and free exercise clauses of the First Amendment (Schaler, 2000). Several states have ruled in favor of the plaintiff pointing out that AA meets the court's criteria of a religious activity, and becomes an "extension" of the state when citizens are ordered into AA. Another problem masquerading as a solution in AA is the idea that believing one is weak, helpless and powerless can build an individual's self-efficacy.

Contrary to what some critics have said about Szasz, he was not an anti-psychiatrist (Szasz, 2009). Szasz repeatedly asserted that he believed in psychiatry between consenting adults. He criticized institutional psychiatry, that is, the union of psychiatry or medicine with the state. Familiar and long-lived religious denominations often call newer sects, even nontraditional offshoots of their own denomination, cults. Critics have denounced what they term "the cult of Thomas Szasz." Again, this is an example of how calling a group a cult is a way of stigmatizing the group and its members (Goffman, 1963; Kaufmann, 1973). The purpose of scapegoating is to expunge evil and affirm the dominant ethic. This is as true today as it was during the time of the Spanish Inquisition (Szasz, 1970).

As mentioned earlier, the cult occupies a place in a member's life similar to the place that most ordinary religions occupy in their members' lives. The group and the beliefs or ideas that bind them together, become a central focus, and rituals based on the ideas may be a frequent activity of members. Disagreement with the beliefs of the group is often

143

penalized, if not punished. Again, the overriding rule of a cult is this: Thou shalt not disagree.

It seems reasonable to associate with others because they share certain beliefs, and it may sometimes be appropriate to exclude those who do not share those beliefs. An association of black police officers appears to have a right to exclude white police officers. Since the cult seeks to eliminate the difference between the individual and the collective, when a conforming individual is criticized by a cult "outsider," the group as a whole feels threatened. The cult experiences the nonbeliever as a threat or danger to the integrity of the group.

When individual members challenge the group ideology, they may eventually be asked to leave. This is the very opposite of what one might imagine an ideal academic environment to be, that is, an environment where disagreement is not only well tolerated but encouraged. Again in truly scientific endeavors, people are constantly trying to disprove current theories. Within academia there are groups with shared beliefs, such as a Marxist or a Catholic group of professors. However, academic freedom stipulates that different viewpoints are not only to be protected, they are invited, encouraged, and welcomed. Not so for the groups we call cults. College psychology departments are notorious for excluding those who take apart the ideas of the majority. Teaching Szasz's ideas to psychology students is an anathema likely to result in being ostracized from the faculty, or excluded from enjoying the liberty of academic freedom.

Many groups we ordinarily do not think of as cults share the beliefs and behaviors people unhesitatingly criticize as cults. So being a cult is an ideal type, and its application a matter of degree. Examples of cults may include institutional psychiatry, the Church of Scientology, Alcoholics Anonymous, Gestalt Therapy guilds, est, Lifespring, and other schools of personality theory, psychoanalysis and related psychodynamic schools of personality based on the idea that there is such a thing as the unconscious mind which can make people behave involuntarily. These groups intensively discourage nonconformity within the membership of adherents (see Rosen, 1978).

Families in Distress

Some people are distressed when a family member or friend gets involved with a cult. This could be a son's involvement with AA, or involvement with an orthodox sect of Judaism, the Hasidim, or whatever. Often those seeking meaning in a cult come from a dysfunctional family, where they were very unhappy. However, a family member who joins a cult is often not viewed as choosing to join the group, that is, joining is considered involuntary. They were tricked into "joining." The contradiction is obvious. A personality change—"he is just not the same person"—is often used to justify viewing the member's involvement as nonvoluntary, "there must be something wrong with him, with his brain, with his mind, with his emotions." In fanciful accounts, the cult allegedly casts a spell on its victims. It allegedly puts them in a trance where they will do whatever the members of a cult tell them to do.

People who leave a cult often say they were taken advantage of by the cult. This is one way they avoid taking responsibility for their behavior and consequences. They are viewed as victims by themselves and others. They blame their indiscretions on powerful others. They view their past misjudgments as actions done to them, not actions they committed or take responsibility for. Parents and others may turn to cult "deprogrammers," in line with this anticult doctrine that people who join did not make a free choice to do so. Parents often don't like the choices their children make, especially when their children stray from the lifestyle and values of parents, and they may also hold the theory that no normal person, or no kin of theirs, would ever make these kinds of choices. Cult deprogrammers are paid to kidnap a friend or family member away from the cult and convert them out of their cult-fashioned trance back into their precult self—a free thinking, individual person who sees the harm in the actions of cult members, one who reembraces the majority view, and eschews the beliefs of the cult.

Are Cults Dangerous?

Many people believe that cults are dangerous. This varies based on social acceptance. The socially unacceptable group is often considered dangerous and bad. The socially acceptable group is considered safe and good. Parents intent on making sure their daughter identifies and practices the religion she grew up with are going to be upset if she believes in an ideology that contradicts that of her parents. They may think that being a member of the cult is going to injure the well-being of their adult child. For example, a Catholic parent may not mind if their child becomes a totally nonpracticing Catholic, or even marries a Protestant, but may be alarmed if their child becomes a Scientologist or a Jehovah's Witness. Today, most any American who grew up as an atheist or in a Judeo-Christian family is going to upset his family of origin if he converts to Islam. Being affiliated with an ideology or an organization is like being affiliated with another person. A parent may object to a child's choice of ideology just as the parent may object to the child's choice of romantic partner.

Parents may be particularly concerned if their child spends time exclusively with the cult, calls it her "family," and acts as though she no longer wants to be associated with her parents. This is a common occurrence. Some cults actually advise that members divorce themselves from their parents, leave their homes and family. Jesus is reported to have said much the same thing (Matthew 10:34–7; Luke 14:26). Cults can be dangerous, in the sense that former associates of the cult member may believe the member is worse off, or in the sense that former cult members themselves come to believe they are worse off. This does not seem dramatically different from many other life choices, such as romantic partners, occupations, or leisure-time activities.

Persuasion Is Different from Coercion

There does not seem to be evidence for the theory that people who join cults are put under a spell or held in some kind of hypnotic trance, aside from anecdotes and hearsay. Observers who jump to such conclusions may just underrate the power of ordinary persuasion and the susceptibility of people to sudden "conversion" to a radically different worldview. Persuasion and coercion are different. The only legal form of coercion is that practiced by the state against citizens who break the law, and parents concerned about the welfare of their children. If a person coerces another person a crime has been committed. Do people in cults do bad things to themselves and others? Sometimes, yes. The "People's Temple Christian Church," run by Pastor Jim Jones, engaged in "mass suicide" (which was in part really "mass murder") in Guyana in 1978. The "Heaven's Gate" cult also engaged in group suicide. These are, of course, exceptional cases, and most cults do not lead to avoidable deaths of members.

The cult of institutional psychiatry commits people innocent of a crime to a mental institution because they allegedly believe they can predict whether said individual is going to harm self or others. As asserted earlier, no one can predict who is going to hurt self or others with an accuracy beyond that expected by chance. That is a fact, not a theory. Despite the fact the United States Supreme Court has upheld the constitutionality of involuntary commitment, it seems obvious to this and other writers that involuntary commitment violates our constitutional entitlement to due process of law. The cult of institutional psychiatry applies its power granted by the state in an arbitrary manner, consistent with the rule of man, not the rule of law. Anyone who comprehends the basics of constitutional law knows what this means. (I have been astounded by the ignorance among psychiatrists when I have lectured on this topic.)

Do people in cults do bad things to themselves and others more than people who are not in cults? We simply don't know. We may judge a particular cult to be harmless or dangerous. One can warn people of the potential consequences of their actions. If they're children under one's care, one can forcibly stop them from doing certain things. If they are adults, they make their own choices, and these may often be quite regrettable, judged by their own best long-term interests. Self-destruction or suicide is as much a right as it is a choice made by a moral agent.

Are People Forced to Join a Cult?

Many people seem to believe that cults coerce people into staying in the group, and physically prevent them from leaving. This did happen in Jim Jones's isolated community, shortly before the "mass suicide." In the television episode of *The Simpsons* devoted to membership in a cult called "Movementarians" (show titled "The Joy of Sect," original airdate February 8, 1998) people were informed they were free to leave, but when they tried to leave, were prevented by armed force. If that happens, it is a criminal act, but among all the thousands of cults, such coercion is rare. Members of cults get into a frame of mind where they fear leaving, they are taught to believe they will be at a loss if the group is not there for them. Some horrible fate will fall upon them should they leave the safety and security of the group. In my many classes on alcoholism and addiction, during which I showed scientific research after research how the loss of control theory of alcoholism and addiction is plain wrong, students of mine who were also in AA were told to drop my class by their AA sponsors, as anything they learned from me that contradicted what they had learned in AA would lead them to become a drunk again and certain death. In fact, when I took issue with the basic ideas supporting belief in the diagnosis and treatment of mental illness in the letters to the editor pages of *The Washington Post*, one psychiatrist wrote in calling me a "murderer" because many people, he asserted, would not seek the help of psychiatrists as a result of reading what I had written. They would die as a result. (He and others did not mention the fact that people were free to seek the assistance of psychologists, social workers, and a large array of secular counselors. Psychiatrists, in my opinion, are notoriously ethnocentric.) Another psychologist in the Washington, DC area, left a message on my telephone answering machine, saying that she and colleagues of hers were going to file a lawsuit against me because many of their patients were coming into their sessions "waving my opinion piece published in the *The Post*" and subsequently quitting psychotherapy. It is psychological dependency and belief in the cult that mainly keeps members from straying.

When members of a cult are presented with contradictory evidence, they tend to move closer to the group, rather than away from it, as common sense would dictate (see Festinger et al., 1956). This is likely due to not wanting to face or admit they had made a bad psychological investment in the beliefs of the group. Psychiatrists who have been led to believe that mental illness really exists are not likely to drop their beliefs and affiliation based on contrary evidence, such as what Szasz has presented. After all they went through a lot of schooling, spent a lot of money, and worked very hard to get to the professional standing they enjoy. They are not pleased to hear that the emperor has no clothes. And they clearly enjoy the power granted to them by the state to put away society's unwanted. (See also Janet Maslin's review of *American heiress: The wild saga of the kidnapping, crimes and trial of Patty Hearst*, by Jeffrey Tobin, New York: Doubleday, 2016. Review dated July 26, 2016, *New York Times Book Review*).

A search on the Internet for opinions regarding the Church of Scientology brings thousands of hits. People claim they were pressured into staying in Scientology, bilked out of thousands of dollars, threatened in all kinds of ways if they go against the group's beliefs. This, again, in my opinion, is all an attempt to simply abdicate responsibility for their actions. People love to blame others for their bad decisions (and take responsibility for their good decisions!). However, evidence that the Church of Scientology committed unlawful acts is sorely lacking. Those are the facts, contrary to claims by those who left the Church of Scientology and blame the Church for enslaving them. People who claim this was the case may report the Church to the police or bring a civil action. It is difficult to find cases where the Church was found liable for unlawful coercion. We can compare this with, for example, the many well-documented cases of pedophilia and sexual abuse by leaders and representatives of the Roman Catholic Church, a body usually defined as not a cult. The Catholic Church is, in my opinion, far more dangerous than the Church of Scientology, especially in regard to the abuse by priests committed against children. After years of fighting with the Department of the Treasury, the federal government recognized the Church of Scientology as a religion and granted it religious status. If people criticized and attacked the Catholic Church the way they criticize and attack the Church of Scientology they would quickly be accused of religious discrimination.

This is not to say that Scientology is ideologically more benign than Catholicism, nor to deny that many people recognize the outrage of the Catholic Church's sex abuse scandals. But the word "cult," applicable to Scientology and not to the Catholic Church, makes all the difference. General denigrations of Judaism are labeled anti-Semitism (Simon & Schaler, 2007), while general denigrations of Scientology are considered unexceptionable.

Identity and Affiliation

People seem to come together and form groups for at least two reasons: They identify and find meaning with the ideology and they feel comfort through companionship and affiliation. In cults, people bind together in various ways and maintain a sense of the herd to avoid being picked off by metaphorical lions (Becker, 1973; Kaufmann, 1973). Whenever a group is threatened, its members huddle closer together. During a crisis, people forget or set aside their differences and work together to face a common enemy ("The enemy of my enemy is my friend," http://www.szasz.com/enemies.html). Individuals form and join groups when their integrity as individuals is threatened. They might just join a group because they agree with it and want to help, too.

"Sharing an identity" means that the members of the group try to think, speak, feel, and behave in a uniform, homogeneous manner. They use the same "thought-terminating clichés," a phrase coined by Robert Jay Lifton in his book of case studies entitled *Thought Reform and the Psychology of Totalism: A Study of "Brainwashing" in China* (1989), that are characteristic of most people in cults (see especially Rosen, 1978). There are people who enjoy ideology more than affiliation, though it is obviously more difficult to avoid social contact if one is learning about ideology from a person, as opposed to a book. Still, the person focused on ideology eschews affiliation and intimacy, is ideology-oriented, and if he is not shy and awkward when it comes to social contact, lacking confidence, he is curmudgeonly, cold and aloof, if not plain antisocial. When people are involved with ideas and groups they may get involved because they like both the ideas and the affiliation, they may shun the ideology and find a sense of family if not community in the social interaction, or vice versa, reject the social interaction and focus as much on ideology and as little on social contact as possible for any number of reasons.

In a group that is labeled a cult, however, the emphasis is more on both ideology and affiliation. Overt or covert rules stipulate that members cannot take one (ideology) and leave the other (affiliation). Affiliation stems from ideology and ideology drives affiliation, if not in the form of proselytizing, that is, trying to recruit new members and converts to both the ideology and the group, then in the process of excluding those who question and doubt the ideology. Ideologically speaking, members of the cult are "yes" men and women. Affiliation-wise, the group is the only group. The rule when it comes to socialization is affiliate only with "us," avoid "them." Many cults insist that members not interact with people outside of the group. Recovering alcoholics in AA should not socialize with people who are not in recovery.

Identity and Contact

When people change their names—not because of marriage—it is usually to try to get away from who they were: it is a primitive way of trying to become a new person by trying to change one's identity. "I am no longer 'Ted' I am 'Jor-el.'" "I am no longer 'Susannah' I am 'Rachel.'" "I am no longer Sara, I am Alex." "I am no longer 'Richard Alpert', I am 'Baba Ram Dass'"—as if one could die and be reborn, become a new person, and escape what was bothersome about a former identity and become someone new. Sometimes a daughter may do this to get away from her parents psychologically, if not physically. This can be a way of creating distance if not separation.

Like it or not, we are each the same person from our birth until our death. We may try to avoid that fact by changing our name and thus our identity, a practice that is more popular than one might imagine. Changing one's name does not necessarily mean that one is denying he is the same person as he was before, but sometimes it does. Someone may just feel that he does not like his original name. John Cheese changed his name to John Cleese. When people join cults they may try to take on a similar new name, a new identity, and try to become a new and different person from who they were prior to their cult life.

When people come together to share an identity as a cult, their personal identity extends to others, and vice versa. This is a major difference from the way people normally relate to one another. Normally, people recognize and respect similarities and differences in personality. Good contact is the appreciation of difference, as F. S. Perls once remarked. There are likes and dislikes, values shared, and differences acknowledged and accepted. Identifying ourselves as individuals is important to good social contact, personal growth, and development. The constancy and clarity of identity, the recognition of differences and similarities, is a key part of maturation and the development of personhood.

Something different happens in the groups that are labeled as cults. Here, people come together seeking to reinforce and strengthen their personal identity through the homogeneity or sameness of identity in the group—everyone in the group strives to be the same, to abolish differences from one another, to think the same way, to speak the same way, to engage in similar behaviors. The cult is decidedly different from other groups in this way. Other groups place a high value on diversity and heterogeneity. The cult is decidedly anti-individualist. When people strive to emphasize their differences, this striving is usually attacked as "egoism," hubris, arrogance, or narcissism—and most importantly, it is usually antithetical to the ideological goals of the cult, be that obedience to the leader, or some state of enlightenment or salvation requiring group cohesiveness. A cult member bows and obeys the guru or leader, if there is one in the cult. He does not bow to himself. As in AA the "higher power" can be anything *but it cannot be the person in recovery himself.* The "higher power" in AA is always another. This is but one way the cult is anti-individualistic (Schaler, 2000).

The difference between a cult and a noncult group is that in cults, the extent to which uniformity exists—both personal and group identity—is much stronger. People are not allowed to question authority if there is a leader. People are not allowed to question the status quo if there is no leader (although some sociologists believe that there is always a leader.)

Radha Soami

During the 1960s and 1970s, many Westerners interested in expanding their consciousness through psychedelic drugs moved away from the drug counter-culture and toward eastern teachers of meditation and mysticism. Young college age American students who became deeply involved with a guru were viewed as having been hypnotized by a cult. This is the image of cult function and following that registered first

151

in peoples' minds then. I want to describe some of the practices of members of this cult now as representative of one with a charismatic leader, consistent with what many people imagine a cult to be. After a discussion of other characteristics of a group that is a cult, I discuss Alcoholics Anonymous, as an example of a leaderless cult.

An interesting, very large yet low-profile cult is the school of Hindu-based mystical practice in the Sikh tradition called Sant Mat (translated means "Saints' Way"), also known as Radha Soami Satsang Beas. (Cf. http://www.rssb.org/ & http://www.scienceofthesoul.org/). Radha Soami means "lord of the soul." The international headquarters called "the Dera" is in the Punjab region of India, about an hour by car from Amritsar, home of the "Golden Temple." There are literally millions of initiates into what is called "The Path." The group is relatively well known in India, and while adherents are scattered throughout the world, many Westerners do not know about it as the group eschews prosyletizing. Initiation, where "seekers" are given meditation instructions, is completely free. As of this time, 2017, there are well over one million initiates.

Many American psychiatrists, psychologists, lawyers, and educated people—the past guru, Maharaj Charan Singh Ji was an Indian lawyer, highly educated, disenchanted with the religion there were born into, were drawn to this cult as well as people from all walks of life as it seemed to be the "safest" relationship with a spiritual leader, and the essence of all religions. While it appears similar to Sikhism, it is different in that the group depends on a living guru, or teacher, also referred to as a "living Master." Past gurus, such as those Sikh gurus following the life of Guru Nanak, will not do, according to Sant Mat. Adherents or disciples of the guru are encouraged to stay in the religion they were raised in as they practiced two forms of very serious meditation and devotion to the guru.

The Lomi School, now the Lomi School Foundation, Inc., centered in California just north of San Francisco, a major force in humanistic psychology, served in the 1970s as one of many unofficial gateways into the Radha Soami cult. The psychiatrist, psychologist, and other mental health counselors leading psychotherapy, "Lomi Body Work" (the first offshoot of "Rolfing," also known as Structural Integration), and "body awareness" programs and sessions at the Lomi School's residential work-shops spoke extensively about their experiences with the guru there, as well as the philosophy of "The Path," and at times what seemed to be the magical powers of the guru. As a result, many of their psychotherapy patients were deeply intrigued by their stories about being with the guru then, Maharaj Charan Singh Ji, now deceased, in India and on his visits to the United States. Their patients became "initiated" into the cult, were told they were going to be reincarnated no more than four more times as a human being, and that the guru, a god-man, would watch over and guide them throughout this life and possibly three other incarnations to eventual god realization. The only requirements for receiving initiation and meditation instruction were abstention from alcohol and mind-altering drugs, no sexual relations before or outside of marriage, and commitment to two and a half hours of meditation daily. The guru could allegedly tell who was spiritually ready to be initiated and who was not, even when the guru was a great distance away, thus, not everyone who applied for initiation would be accepted.

The leaders of the Lomi School were very attractive, handsome and beautiful men and women, each married, each initiated by the current Master of Sant Mat, and each highly skilled as psychiatrist, psychologist, and various types of counselors. They used their presentation of self to lure their patients into what some would call transference, others might call submission, and still others refer to as psychological dependency. They had the sing-song hypnotic and rhythmical voice that many leaders of cults use to draw people in. Their families were often brought in to observe patients working on themselves in group Gestalt Therapy. The rule of no dual relationships, taken seriously by professional psychologically oriented practitioners in their code of ethics, was deeply muddled by the leaders at the Lomi School. Sexual contact was made between patients and therapists, especially among those people they trained as Lomi Body Workers, and a code of ethics guarding against dual relationships was rejected by the founders. Formally trained in their brand of physical therapy, or the first offshoot of Rolfing, I wrote the first ethical code, fed up with what I considered unethical activity on the part of practititioners, as well as their trainers, and I was told that a code of ethics, penalties, and dismissal of therapists from the organization was not needed. I was belittled and ridiculed for writing and requesting that a code of ethics be required,and as a result, I resigned from the organization when the code of ethics was rejected. Years later a minimal code of ethics apparently was adopted. I ceased all contact with the organization prior to then, and I have no idea as to its current status. The blurring of lines between professional responsibility as therapist, unofficial spiritual leaders and conduits for Sant Mat, and blatant sexual relationships was more than a little obvious.

The Cult of Radha Soami Satsang Beas

Many years ago when I was about 26 years old, I stayed for several weeks at the Radha Soami Satsang Beas in Beas, Punjab district, India. The stay was free and I was treated well. I had ample opportunity to engage with the guru there, Maharaj Charan Singh Ji, and I seized that opportunity. I often took issue with what the guru said, and challenged his assertions. The two of us bantered and talked over one another as the exchange became at times more passionate.

It is important to realize that this guru was and subsequent ones are regarded by followers as both god and man simultaneously, the way Jesus and Buddha were regarded. I enjoyed my experience there immensely, I had received "initiation" a few years previously and practiced ways of life suggested including lactovegetarianism and meditation. I left that group after engaging the guru, and returning home to my wife and three-year-old daughter, the one thing that occurred there clearly supported my understanding of cults. I realized that this group, and its leader, for all their good intentions, qualified as a cult.

There are often ritual ways of greeting and leaving people that those in cults abide by. In the Radha Soami Satsang cult, with headquarters based in Beas, India, and millions of disciples around the world, initiated by a "living Master" or "Satguru," disciples greet and say goodbye to each other by holding their hands together as if in prayer, bowing, and saying "Radha Soami." It is always expected that the persons present who did not say "Radha Soami" first will say it in response. If the other does not respond with "Radha Soami," something peculiar in the interaction has occurred. Those who do not say it may be treated with suspicion. They have broken an unspoken rule of ritual interaction.

After I argued with the guru several evenings, and this occurred in front of several hundred Westerners in what was called the "Western Guest House," people came up and lambasted me for taking issue with the guru. They said one should never disagree or argue with "the Master." I replied that I had traveled many thousands of miles to converse with him, and I would say whatever I felt like saying. Those comments of theirs reinforced my ideas regarding agreement and disagreement. Disagreeing with the guru was forbidden among adherents.

I do want to point out that these sentiments regarding disagreement were those of adherents, disciples, called "satsangis," not the guru himself. The guru welcomed disagreement and was very gracious toward me. Interestingly he seemed very different from his followers. The contradiction, the Orwellian "doublethink" was this: He was considered simultaneous human and not human. That was the ultimate contradiction that seemed to be a key to confusion on the part of followers. Another impossible test of the cult was this: Adherents were told by the guru and other adherents that the meditation and way of life was a "science." Of course, nothing could be further from the truth. If we look back to what both Feynman and Popper said about science, we clearly see the missing pieces here. Falsification was impossible in the Radha Soami cult. People may well have invested in years of meditation in the work on the Path. It was considered a science in that by practicing the meditation and rules of conduct, vegetarianism, no drugs or alcohol consumption, no sex before or outside of marriage, the disciples would experience various states of higher consciousness, mainly through meditation. I told disciples that I had practiced all that was suggested to me, and the result was that I had none of the experiences promised. When I asked why that was, I was told that I had not practiced hard enough. If I practiced longer hours of meditation, the inner experiences of higher consciousness would be experienced. I did what was suggested and I still had none of the experiences others claimed I would have. Again I was told that I had to practice longer. Obviously this was simply a way to keep an adherent in the group. There was never a possibility of falsification. Anyone could leave the group and practice at any time. These were all, in my opinion, examples of doublethink, contradiction.

I investigated other groups when I returned from India to find out more about the role of doublethink and cults generally. I had heated arguments with close friends who I believed cast a blind eye toward blatant contradiction, tautology, and nonsensical thinking. To my chagrin, those previously important friendships ended. For example, in Alcoholics Anonymous, people said to be addicted due to a disease could not use their will to stop drinking. However, they are told to use their will to stop drinking! Moreover, people are regarded as having the disease called alcoholism before they ever took a drink of alcohol, and for untold years after they had become sober.

Other rules of the cult include the requirement that adherents are not allowed to affiliate with those outside of the group. Some groups lay down rules about who members may associate with, others do not. This is a matter of degree. In the cult we are speaking of the extreme. There is strong inclusiveness in the cult—members are deeply committed to both their ideology and the group—and exclusiveness—members are deeply committed to excluding and avoiding those who disagree with or challenge their ideology, unless they see an opportunity to convert others. The attempt to bring in new members strengthens the cultists' resolve regarding the value of the group. This is a balancing act. While this is frequently a characteristic of many normal groups, again in the cult it is much stronger.

Brainwashed?

When a charismatic leader holds the group together, the leader "lives life for the members." This way he suffers the difficulties of interaction with the outside world, something that his followers may find intolerable, and is paid in return with devotion and worship. Never underestimate the effect of bowing and loyalty to the guru. People in the cult begin to believe and claim that he has superpowers and is more than human. When people think of cult members as in a "trance," they usually mean that cult members have been "brainwashed" or hypnotized, tricked, by a charismatic leader, someone who is often exceptionally insightful about human nature, behavior, and experience. The leader may often have a very attractive, rhythmical, musical quality to the way he speaks, to both disciples and outsiders (potential recruits). This makes him and the group especially attractive. Members in leaderless cults act similarly toward one another. Their use of language, metaphors, adjectives and adverbs, is strikingly similar.

Because cult members are said to be in a trance, most people believe that it is very difficult for them to break out of the cult, to free themselves and act independent of the group or leader that seeks to control them. This is why deprogrammers kidnap the cult member and try to turn him around through deprogramming messages. The process is not unlike what goes on in the cult itself. Persuasion is useless. Coercion, according to deprogrammers, is necessary to get the person away from the cult.

When we use the word "brainwashed," we may think of the movie *The Manchurian Candidate* (1962), starring Frank Sinatra (and remade recently, 2004). In that movie people were captured and hypnotized by the Communist Chinese to assassinate American political leaders at a later date—posthypnotic suggestion. Obviously, "brainwash" is a metaphor. The term refers to a trance-like, hypnotic state of consciousness where a person is allegedly awake and simultaneously asleep. The movie was fiction, and it lent itself to the idea that the Communists could infiltrate America by hypnotizing Americans. The movie came out at the time of a "Red Scare" in American politics: Joe McCarthy had launched a pogrom of sorts accusing people of being a communist in ways reminiscent of accusations concerned witchcraft (See especially Arthur Miller's *The Crucible*, 1955).

McCarthy made a political issue of the lists of government employees who had been identified as security risks without anything being done. He accepted there was nothing illegal in being a communist and that everyone had a perfect right to be a communist. However, government employees who came in contact with classified information were asked if they were communists, because it was understood that they would pass any information on to Moscow. If a government employee denied being a communist when he was a communist, this could be grounds for disciplinary action, including dismissal. Similarly today, if a government employee had connections with "ISIS," we would immediately launch all sorts of CIA protocols.

Lifton's *Thought Reform and the Psychology of Totalism* was influential for popular beliefs concerning trance states and cults. He identifies personality characteristics of people who did not recover well from thought reform. The book also became popular as the deprogrammer's bible. The locus classicus for this mind control is *Trilby* by George du Maurier (1894), though in that case there was no "organization," but simply a controlling person whose name became a symbol of such controllers: Svengali.

Cults and Personality

The stronger an individual's confidence in self, the less likely an individual will succumb to demands for cult conformity, again based on Lifton's findings and analysis. Individuals with a strong sense of personal autonomy are less likely to become involved in cults. If they do become involved in a cult, they are more likely to recover from the cult experience in a way that preserves a strong sense of self (compared to those whose self-concept was considerably weaker prior to the cult experience). What is also likely to be true is that individuals with a strong sense of self are less likely to feel threatened when cult members attack them. Moreover, individuals eschewing cult affiliation may elicit resentment from true believers (Kaufmann, 1973).

Based on Lifton's analysis of those recovering from Communist Chinese thought reform prisons, individuals with backgrounds involving chronic identity confusion, excessive guilt, and "totalistic" or dichotomous thinking, appear to experience more difficulty in reestablishing

157

themselves in their post-thought reform camp life, compared to those individuals with a clearer sense of identity, less guilt, and a more accurate sense of psychological perspective. Individuals exhibiting a strong sense of personal autonomy appear more resistant to criticism directed at them by a group of individuals at odds with their particular ideology. To me, it appears that those persons with the characteristics that Lifton found, are more likely to join and involve themselves in cult experiences. Those with identity confusion, particularly during their adolescent years, excessive guilt, and totalistic or dichotomous thinking are more likely to join a cult, be it leaderless or with a leader.

In clinical hypnosis, the hypnotist and subject pretend their wills are confluent with one another. The subject, theoretically, does not have a say in the process, once the hypnosis begins. He abdicates responsibility for his behavior. The sense of ego separateness between the two is purposely obscured by the hypnotist and the subject. In analysis and psychotherapy generally, this experience is called "transference." As long as the client in either hypnosis or psychotherapy maintains an acute awareness of self, that is, he persists in appreciating the difference between self and environment, a point referred to as the "ego boundary" by Perls (1947), the hypnosis and transference game will fail. In fact, a goal of good therapy or analysis is to achieve this state of autonomy. As Szasz has pointed out in conversations elsewhere, when asked what he considered to be "good therapy," he responded: Any therapy or analysis that helps a person achieve personal autonomy and independence is good therapy. Szasz never defined, described, or offered instruction in psychotherapy or psychoanalysis beyond that. He considered the fact that he did not found another school of psychology or psychotherapy to be one of his major accomplishments. A person cannot merge his mind with another, anymore than he can merge his body with another. Some schools of psychotherapy may view this as an obstruction to good therapy, others view it as a means to achieving success (Szasz, 1965).

Good contact and a hypnotic trance are opposing states of consciousness. Thus, good contact antidotes a trance state. Moreover, good contact between therapist and client is not contingent upon cultivating transference, contrary to what many analysts who believe in an unconscious mind say. Psychotherapy fails when the client chooses to see the therapist as someone other than he really is, and when therapists encourage clients to see them as someone other than who they really are. The conversation called psychotherapy can be successful to facilitating deep personality change when a client sees the therapist as a struggling and fallible human being himself. These assumptions are based on the premise that the goal of psychotherapy is achieving individual autonomy. This means seeing the analyst as a human being engaged in his own existential struggles.

An extreme example of this ability to resist hypnosis and brain-washing is seen in the movie *The Ipcress File* (1965). By deliberately pressing a metal nail into his hand actor Michael Caine used his experience of pain to force an awareness of self. He avoided listening to the hypnotic voice of an "other," an "other" seeking to make Caine's will confluent with his own—against Caine's will. Caine's character found a way to maintain autonomy in the face of that psychological coercion. He was able to fight the psychological influence of another intent on dictating a particular self-concept. The point intended here is that by focusing on himself in such a way, he was able to resist the attempt by the other to force a psychological merge—a merge that is coerced by one onto another. The force intent on hypnotizing Caine is not dissimilar to the persuasion tactics of proselytizing cult members in the extreme. While typically cult members do not undergo anything like the extreme physical torture and enforced physical disorientation of the character Harry Palmer, played by Michael Caine, I believe that studying and familiarizing oneself with the extreme can assist with comprehending what goes on in milder cults intolerant of difference of opinion.

Breaking up the Group

There are ways of applying these ideas to individuals under the "spell cast by others" (Becker, 1973). One way of testing the cult nature of a group is by challenging the ideology binding the group together. We can discover something about the nature of a group by how well its members tolerate opposition to the ideology holding the group together. How well do members tolerate difference of opinion, opinion that challenges the very ideological heart of the group?

Members of the cult are like a colony of insects when disturbed. A frenzy of activity and protective measures are executed when core ideologies are challenged. The stronger the evidence challenging the truthfulness of the group ideology, the more likely members of the cult are to either lash out in a more or less predictable fashion, fall apart, or disband into separate cult colonies. Alcoholics Anonymous has often been characterized as a cult, and this generally involves a derogatory judgment (AA) (Kurtz, 1988; Antze, 1987; Leach & Norris, 1977).

AA: A Leaderless Cult

What follows now is the result of interactions with members of AA and the author. I presented scientific arguments and conclusions testing and falsifying the "loss of control theory" of alcoholism, the cornerstone upon which the disease concept rests. People in AA use the "loss of control theory" as a unifying ideology and identity. If people wrote they had a disease, I wrote that disease is different from behavior. In other words I disagreed with the various claims that held the group of AA together. While mainly those who have been coerced by government into attending AA based on criminal infractions while intoxicated, mostly drunken driving, AA is also often viewed as a harmless and perhaps highly beneficial social service group with no specific religious or other doctrinal peculiarities. Those who hold the scientifically unsupported position that addiction is a disease characterized by loss of control generally look more favorably upon AA. If AA works at all, and there is convincing evidence that it is no more effective than leaving people to their own devices, it is probably through the sense of community that helps (Schaler, 2000). In other words, some people manage to stabilize their lives through their experience with AA. A positive community experience was likely missing for many people prior to being in AA.

However, there is extensive evidence to show that AA is no more effective than no treatment, and in other studies AA is no more effective than a form of treatment known as motivational enhancement (focused on strengthening self-efficacy) and cognitive behavioral therapy (focused on recognizing and changing one's irrational thoughts to rational ones) (see the discussion of Vaillant's work, and Project MATCH, in Schaler, 2000). In other words, it makes little difference whether one goes into the best paid, contemporary psychological treatment has to offer. The bottom line is that treatment is as effective as no treatment at all, that is, leaving people to their own devices.

Encounters between those who consider AA a cult and those who do not, as well as whether addiction is a choice versus a disease, can become heated at times (for example, Madsen et al., 1990; Goodwin & Gordis, 1988; Schaler, 2000). Exchanges documented here occurred on the editorial pages of large and small newspapers, live radio-talk shows, scientific journals, local political settings, and in the past eighteen years or so in discussion groups on the Internet.

It is a mistake to attribute the nature of critical response solely to a personal way of showing that the cult's ideology is illogical. People critical of cults, more so their ideology, present their ideas in sensitive and tactful ways and they have met with similar forms of denunciation and character assassination, the typical form of rebuttal. *Ad hominem* rebuttals are the standard (Fingarette, 1989; Peele, 1992; Searles, 1993; Madsen, 1989; Wallace, 1993a, 1993b).

While many of the following studies may seem dated, their truthfulness, in my opinion, never goes out of date. I believe it is a mistake to deny a study because it is five years old. AA stays the same. Much evidence has been adduced to support the view that AA is a cult. Greil and Rudy (1983) studied conversion to the world view of AA and reported that

> [t]he process by which individuals affiliate with A.A. entails a radical transformation of personal identity in that A.A. provides the prospective affiliate not merely with a solution to problems related to drinking, but also with an overarching world view with which the convert can and must reinterpret his or her past experience. . . . Our analysis suggests that the central dynamic in the conversion process is coming to accept the opinions of reference others. (p. 6).

> [I]t appears . . . that contact with A.A. is more likely to be accompanied by a greater degree of coercion than . . . most cases of religious conversion. (1983, p. 23)

Alexander and Rollins (1984) described how Lifton's (1961) eight brainwashing techniques used by the Communist Chinese operate in AA. "[T]he authors contend that AA uses all the methods of brain washing, which are also the methods employed by cults" (Alexander & Rollins, 1984, p. 45).

Galanter (1989) has written a lot on the topic of cults:

> As in the Unification Church workshops, most of those attending AA chapter meetings are deeply involved in the group ethos, and the expression of views opposed to the group's model of treatment is subtly or expressly discouraged. A good example is the fellowship's response to the concept of controlled drinking, an approach to alcoholism treatment based on limiting alcohol intake rather than totally abstaining. Some investigators and clinicians have reported success with this alternative to treatment. The approach, however, is unacceptable within the AA tradition, and the option is therefore anathema to active members. It is rarely brought up by speakers at meetings and suppressed when it is raised . . . (Galanter, 1989, p. 185)

Sadler (1977) writes to that effect when she stated that

> AAers seek a relationship with the supernatural in order to cease managing their own lives. . . . AA . . . tells the newcomer that his life is unmanageable and that it is ridiculous for him to try to manage it. . . . By deliberately denying the ability to control their lives, AAers' former drunken situations are brought under control. . . . Most importantly, abstinence is not considered a kind of control. The individual who comes to AA in order to control his drinking will be disappointed. AAers insist that abstinence is possible only when powerlessness is conceded. AA offers supportive interaction in which powerlessness comes to be positively valued. (Sadler, 1977, p. 208)

What follows here is again based on my own experience interacting with members of an Internet listserv devoted to AA. When ideas regarding voluntariness, responsibility, and addiction are introduced to members of AA and devout adherents to the disease concept of addiction, people who are usually involved with AA in some way, the following responses are likely to occur:

Name-calling

The person introducing ideas that are taboo to the cult (here referred to as the heretic, critic, or writer) is belittled and laughed at. Derogatory comments are leveled. Name calling often ensues, for example, the writer was called a "thoughtless dweeb," told "you are your own worst enemy," that the writer was a "crackpot psychologist," a "fascist," "doctor baby," an "arrogant son of a bitch," "contemptible," "immature for a guy with a Dr. before his name," and a person engaging in "highly unscientific behavior," who has embarked on a "personal vendetta."

This is behavior common to other cults as well as AA, where one disagrees with the ideology. More important, when one points out the contradiction in the way members of the cult think, the response is at times ferocious. It is this upset among cult members when the contradictory nature of their thinking—the doublethink referred to by Orwell—is exposed that elicits the angriest response. AA has set itself up for this kind of scrutiny, however, by involving itself directly in the professional treatment world, instead of remaining separate from the courts and medicine the way many religious organizations prefer.

Accusations of Murder

After the initial mocking and belittling, the criticism of the heretic appears to take a more serious turn. The ideas presented by the critic are considered potentially dangerous. People who do not know better will misuse them and kill themselves or others. Thus, the critic should be held accountable for murder, or the death of another. The heretic then personifies evil in the eyes of cult members. It is at this point that the exchange could become physically dangerous to the critic.

You're Only in It for the Money

The heretic may also be accused at this point of having an economic investment in his particular point of view. For example, the writer has been accused of trying to pirate potential psychotherapy clients away from AA.

Diagnosis of Mental Illness

Another tack the cult members often take is to accuse the heretic of being mentally ill. Psychiatric diagnosis is frequently used as a weapon. The taboo ideas are alleged to stem from personal trauma the heretic has not dealt with, and his statements in opposition to the group ideology are considered projections, the function of "denial," an unconscious process that is said to be a symptom of his mental illness. When people get very angry with someone, they often psychoanalyze and diagnose them.

It Takes One to Know One

The critic's ideas about AA may be termed invalid because he or she is not a drug addict. This is often asserted without knowing the facts. The heretic may very well have been what others call an "addict" or "alcoholic." Frequently, the critic is asked, "have you ever had a drug problem?" Whereas in the "diagnosis of mental illness" case the motive driving apparent concern is that the critic's inappropriate behavior is likely to stem from a mental illness, in this case, if the heretic has not had a drug problem or shared in the problems-of-living experienced by cult members, he or she is said to be incapable of speaking from legitimate experience, as it is only by this experience that someone can "know" what the truth is regarding their cult ideology. If he says he has been in trouble with drugs or alcohol, then he is apparently having a relapse, evidenced by his "denial" through defense mechanisms called "rationalization," "intellectualization"—or what is referred to in AA as "stinkin' thinkin."

Invoking Authority

A demand for scientific evidence to support the heretical ideas always emerges. In AA, members often cite scientific findings to support their claims regarding involuntariness. That certain medical organizations have endorsed their ideology is brought forth as evidence of the veracity of their ideas. When scientific evidence to the contrary is presented by the critic, the research is said to be too old to be valid, not extensive enough, subject to diverse interpretations, and ultimately no match for personal experience. At times, when scientific information is brought into the discussion by the critic, other scientists will accuse the heretic of unethical use of knowledge and influence, and threaten to report him or her to some professional association in hopes that he or she may become professionally censored.

Shaming

The assault on the heretic is based on the idea that facts are cruel and insensitive to people who have done him no harm. "Is this the way you treat your friends (or patients)?"

The counterargument to the heretic can then involve scientific and philosophical reductionism to the point that few, if any, conclusions regarding the issues at hand can ever be reached. Circuitous arguments evolve. Blatant contradictions emerge, for example, "the alcoholic cannot willfully control his drinking, therefore, he must be abstinent." Yet, people choose to abstain from drinking alcoholic beverage. The alcoholic allegedly cannot choose to control his drinking, therefore, he must choose to control his drinking. Henderson (1984) offers a graphic example of the misuse of analogy, in a conversation where an AA counselor likened alcoholism to diarrhea.

Recovering from the Cult

For some, these confrontations are enough to shake them out of their cult daze, arouse their curiosity, and assist in getting them to leave the group. Occasionally, a member of the cult may yield suddenly to the critic, attempting to practice a "turn the other cheek" portion of the ideological doctrine. If a personal dialogue can be achieved and continued between a cult member and the heretic an emotional catharsis may occur for the cultist and this can become a major event in breaking the hypnotic spell, admitting that the person was pretending to be in a trance.

Humor is useful in further diffusing volatile contacts, along with divulging of personal information on the part of the heretic. Those intent on preserving the cult will often go underground and avoid any contact with the heretic whatsoever. In the end, if the cult member can recognize the price he pays in terms of his own integrity and autonomy by sacrificing his individuality, he will leave the group, forgive himself and others in the group, and learn a valuable lesson from the cult experience.

Some Concluding Thoughts

In conclusion, as we have seen here, the conventional meaning and descriptions of cults can as easily be applied to socially acceptable groups, as it can to socially unacceptable groups. Groups that may be considered cults emphasize a strong unifying identity and philosophy to hold the group together. Cults can have a leader or be leaderless. There is no evidence to show that people are "brainwashed" and/or coerced into a cult. Persuasion is different from coercion, and what people claim is coercion is persuasion. The number one rule of cults is "thou shalt not disagree."

The more a unifying philosophy can be challenged and disproved, or falsified—In other words, the more a group allows for difference of opinion, the less likely the group as cult is likely to serve destructive interests. While academic and educational experience in general, specifically emphasizing academic freedom, and freedom of speech for both students and faculty/administrators is clearly essential to constructive human development, it is also essential to becoming an autonomous person as well as a true producer, and essential to developing and ultimately experiencing self-actualization, as Walter Kaufmann (1973) described autonomy in his important book entitled *Without guilt and justice* a work, in my opinion, very consistent with Thomas Szasz's writings, as well as Becker's (1973) writings and Leifer's writings on the meaning of heroism. In fact, Szasz told me once how much he admired Kaufmann. The more freedom to disagree in state mandated treatment programs for addiction and the putative treatment of mental illness, the better for all involved. This is consistent with our First Amendment rights, that is, our right to freedom of expression. Cults equal the absence of this kind of freedom. Worried that I had upset too many people through my published writings, I remember saying to Tom, "perhaps I should curb the things I say." "That," he retorted, "is the last thing you should do, Jeff!"

References

Alexander, B. K. (1987). The disease and adaptive models of addiction: A framework evaluation. *Journal of Drug Issues, 17,* 47–66.

Alexander, B. K. (1990). The empirical and theoretical bases for an adaptive model of addiction. *Journal of Drug Issues, 20,* 37–65.

Alexander, F., & Rollins, M. (1984). Alcoholics anonymous: The unseen cult. *California Sociologist: A Journal of Sociology and Social Work, Winter,* 33–48.

Antze, P. (1987). Symbolic action in alcoholics anonymous. In Mary Douglas, (Ed.), *Constructive drinking: Perspectives on drink from anthropology* (pp. 149–181). New York: Cambridge University Press.

Barrett, W. (1979). *The illusion of technique: A search for meaning in a technological civilization.* New York: Anchor.

Becker, E. (1973). *The denial of death.* New York: Free Press.

Berger, L. (1991). *Substance abuse as symptom: A psychoanalytic critique of treatment approaches and the cultural beliefs that sustain them.* Hillsdale, NJ: The Analytic Press.

Festinger, L, Riecken, H. W., & Schacter, S. (1956). When prophecy fails: A social and psychological study of a modern group that predicted the destruction of the world. New York: Harper-Torchbooks.

Feynman, R. (1974). Caltech's commencement address. http://calteches .library.caltech.edu/51/2/CargoCult.htm

Fingarette, H. (1988). Heavy drinking: The myth of alcoholism as a disease. Berkeley, CA: University of California Press.

Fingarette, H. (1989). A rejoinder to Madsen. *The Public Interest, 95,* 118–121.

Freud, S. (1959). *Group psychology and analysis of the ego.* New York: Norton.

Galanter, M. (1989). *Cults: Faith, healing, and coercion.* New York: Oxford University Press.

Goffman, E. (1963). *Stigma: Notes on the Management of Spoiled Identity.* New York: Simon & Schuster.

Goodwin, F. K., Gordis, E, et al. (1988, November 5). Alcoholism most certainly is a disease. *The Washington Post,* A21.

Greil, A. L., & Rudy, D. R. (1983). Conversion to the world view of alcoholics anonymous: A refinement of conversion theory. *Qualitative Sociology, 6,* 5–28.

Henderson, C. D. (1985). Countering resistance to acceptance of denial and the disease concept in alcoholic families: Two examples of experiential teaching. *Alcoholism Treatment Quarterly, 1,* 117–121.

Kaufmann, W. (1973). *From decidophobia to autonomy without guilt and justice.* New York: Delta.

Kurtz, E. (1988). *AA: The story (A Revised Edition of Not- God: A History of Alcoholics Anonymous).* New York: Harper & Row.

Leach, B., & Norris, J. L. (1977). Factors in the development of Alcoholics Anonymous (A.A.). In Benjamin Kissin & Henri Begleiter (Eds.), *Treatment and rehabilitation of the chronic alcoholic: The biology of alcoholism* (Vol. 5, pp. 441–543). New York: Plenum Press.

Lifton, R. J. (1961). *Thought reform and the psychology of totalism: A study of "brainwashing" in China.* New York: Norton.

Madsen, W. (1989). Thin thinking about heavy drinking. *The Public Interest,* 95, 112–118.

Madsen, W, Berger, D., & Bremy, F. (1990). Alcoholism a myth? *Skeptical Inquirer: Journal of the Committee for the Scientific Investigations of the Paranormal, 14*(Summer), 440–442.

Miller, A. (1955). *The crucible.* New York: Bantam

Orwell, G. (1981). *Nineteen-eighty four* (pp. 176–178). New York: New American Library.

Peele, S. (1992). Alcoholism, politics, and bureaucracy: The consensus against controlled-drinking therapy in America. *Addictive Behaviors, 17*, 49–62.

Perls, F. S. (1947). *Ego, hunger and aggression: A revision of Freud's theory and method.* London: Allen & Unwin.

Radha Soami Satsang Beas & Sant Mat. No date. Cf. http://www.rssb.org/ and http://www.scienceofthesoul.org/

Reich, W. (1945). *Character analysis.* New York: Farrar, Straus and Giroux.

Rosen, R. D. (1978). *Psychobabble: Fast talk and quick cure in the era of feelings.* New York: Athenum.

Sadler, P. O. (1977). The "crisis cult" as a voluntary association: An interactional approach to alcoholics anonymous. *Human Organization, 36*, 207–210.

Schaler, J. A. (2000). *Addiction is a choice.* Chicago: Open Court.

Searles, J. S. (1993). Science and fascism: Confronting unpopular ideas. *Addictive Behaviors, 18*, 5–8.

Simon, R. J., & Schaler, J. A. (Eds.). (2008). Special issue. Anti-semitism the world over in the twenty-first century. *Current Psychology, 26*(3–4), Special Issue.

Singer, M. T., & Lalich, J. (1995). *Cults in our midst: The hidden menace in our everyday lives.* San Francisco, CA: Jossey-Bass.

Szasz, T. S. (1965). *The ethics of psychoanalysis: The theory and method of autonomous psychotherapy.* New York: Basic Books.

Szasz, T. (1970). *The manufacture of madness: A comparative study of the inquisition and the mental health movement. With a new preface by the author.* Syracue, NY: Syracuse University Press

Szasz, T. (2009). Antipsychiatry: Quackery squared. Syracuse, NY: Syracuse University Press.

Wallace, J. (1993a). Fascism and the eye of the beholder: A reply to J.S. Searles on the controlled intoxication issue. *Addictive Behaviors, 18*, 239–251.

Wallace, J. (1993b). Letters to the editors. *Addictive Behaviors, 18*, 1–4.

West, L. J. (1991). Psychiatry and scientology. Cult Awareness and Information Library. Retrieved from http://www.caic.org.au/index.php?option=com _content&task=view&id=932&Itemid=12. Originally printed in *The Southern California Psychiatrist*, July 1990, pp. 13–16.

8

Schizophrenia, Then and Now: The *Libation Bearers* of Aeschylus

Michael Scott Fontaine

1: *When human life lay foul to see and groveling upon the earth, crushed by the weight of Religion, who showed her face from the realms of heaven, lowering upon mortals with dreadful mien, it was a man of Greece who dared first to raise his mortal eyes to meet her, and first to stand forth to meet her: him neither the stories of the gods nor thunderbolts checked, nor the sky with its revengeful roar, but all the more it spurred the eager daring of his mind . . .*
—Lucretius (c. 99–c. 55 BC), in praise of Epicurus (341–270 BC)[1]

2: *To see what is in front of one's nose needs a constant struggle.*
—George Orwell (1903–50)[2]

3: *They are a blot on all mankind.*
—Arthur Schopenhauer (1788–1860), of the slaveholding states of North America[3]

Readers of Aeschylus' *Libation Bearers*, a Greek tragedy of 458 BC, routinely assert or assume that the hero, Orestes, kills his mother at the behest of the god Apollo. The work of the American psychiatrist Thomas Szasz (1920–2012) shows us why we ought not make that assumption. It thus sets the tragedy in an entirely new light and, if set alongside the evidence of Plautus' *The Menaechmus Brothers*, entails important consequences for the history of (paranoid) schizophrenia in Western society.

Schizophrenia, observed Thomas Szasz, is "the sacred symbol of psychiatry."[4] He was right. It is easy to wonder whether depression is merely a Latin word for sadness, or neurosis merely a Greek name for self-doubt or stupidity (as Szasz, the late medical doctor and professor of psychiatry, referred to it elsewhere). With schizophrenia, by contrast, we move into frightening territory. To the layman, the bizarre behaviors and claims associated with that word do appear to be the outward manifestation of a brain disease; how else could one explain them? Because clinical experience with people labeled schizophrenic is both rare and restricted, we are prone to trust what our acknowledged experts and authorities tell us about the origin of those bizarre behaviors, rather than to trust our own powers of observation and reasoning.[5]

Szasz's existential view of persons labeled schizophrenic is not only more humane than the mechanistic view set forth by neuroscientists. In this paper I would like to show how Szasz's view also revolutionizes the interpretation of the literature of ancient Greece and, in so doing, sets an aspect of the eternal human condition in a new light.

Schizophrenia: Its Alleged Nature and Origin

The scourge of schizophrenia allegedly surrounds us. According to the website of the National Institute of Mental Health (NIMH), this dread disease affects about 1 percent of Americans today—that is, about 3.2 million individuals. NIMH adds that schizophrenia is a chronic, severe, incurable, and disabling brain disorder. According to psychiatrist Nancy Andreasen, who calculates the lifetime prevalence of schizophrenia at 1 percent worldwide, or about 71 million people, "Schizophrenia is a disease of the brain that is expressed clinically as a disease of the mind."[6] Its cause is unknown but most experts assume it is genetic.[7] According to E. Fuller Torrey, M.D., the founder and Executive Director of the Stanley Medical Research Institute and a high-profile schizophrenia researcher, "schizophrenia is caused by changes in the brain. . . . Schizophrenia is thus a disease of the brain in exactly the same sense that Parkinson's disease, multiple sclerosis, epilepsy, and Alzheimer's disease are diseases of the brain."[8] Despite this alleged certainty, no specific gene or allele (genetic mutation) for schizophrenia, and no specific area of the brain, has been identified to differentiate schizophrenic persons from "normals." Scientists cannot differentiate schizophrenics from normals with an accuracy beyond that expected by chance, simply by identifying genetic mutations or abnormal size and function of specific areas of the brain.

Behind the confident rhetoric of Drs. Andreasen and Torrey lies the tacit belief that schizophrenia is a recent arrival to the annals of medicine. According to psychiatry text and reference books, the disease is barely two hundred years old. The first clinical descriptions allegedly date to the year 1809 in London and Paris, after which cases start to sky-rocket.[9] And attempts to find examples of schizophrenia before 1809, especially in the extensive literature of classical antiquity, routinely fail. As one 2003 survey put it, "in ancient Greek and Roman literature, there were no descriptions of individuals with schizophrenia."[10] Two hundred years later, therefore, NIMH's claim that over three million Americans are suffering from schizophrenia today is especially sober-ing when one realizes that in 2009, fewer than 1.2 million Americans were HIV positive.[11]

The sudden appearance and proliferation of schizophrenia has given rise to ongoing debates about whether schizophrenia has always existed under some other guise or whether it really is an epidemic of recent origin, comparable to the outbreaks of syphilis and AIDS; and if it *is* comparable to them, then whether it could be caused by environmental or infectious agents, such as Toxoplasma gondii. (As of 2016, however, no environmental, bacterial, or viral agent has been identified.) The debate is called the "recency vs. persistency hypothe-ses" and the recency hypothesis camp is clearly winning. This explains why researchers worldwide ceaselessly look for physical causes (both genetic and infectious) rather than existential reasons, and why they continue to try different treatments—some of them physical, such as electroconvulsive therapy (ECT), lobotomy, or other forms of surgery, but the majority increasingly chemical applications, especially the use of neuroleptic (or "antipsychotic") drugs—drugs that increase or inhibit the flow of different neurotransmitters.

In this paper I maintain that the entire apparatus on which the recency hypothesis depends is fundamentally wrong. Bolstered by several insights into the human condition bequeathed to us by Thomas Szasz, I do so by challenging an assumption that readers regularly make about an ancient Greek tragedy called *Libation Bearers*.

Aeschylus' Libation Bearers

Libation Bearers is the second play in a trilogy called *The Oresteia*. Written by Aeschylus (c. 525–c. 456 BC), it debuted in Athens' Theater of Dionysus in 458 BC.[12] Long ago as that is, the play is set ever further back in time, in the Bronze Age of c. 1200 BC, and in the Greek city of Argos. The play dramatizes the return to Argos of a legendary hero named Orestes to avenge the murder of his father.

Why has Orestes come home? The first play of Aeschylus' trilogy, called *Agamemnon*, was set ten years before *Libation Bearers*. In it Orestes' father, Agamemnon, is murdered by his mother, Clytemnestra, and her lover, Aegisthus, and together they seize the throne of Argos. At the time, Orestes was a boy of about ten years old, and upon his father's murder his nanny spirits him away to safety. When *Libation Bearers* begins, a decade has passed and today—the day of the play—Orestes has come home for the first time. His age is never stated but he is about 20 years old. With the help of his companion, Pylades, he plans to kill Clytemnestra and Aegisthus. As the action unfolds we watch Orestes disguise himself, penetrate the palace defenses, and—at the climax— strike the couple down with a sword, one by one, in cold blood. The play's chorus of citizen women—the "libation bearers" of the title—hails him as their liberator and savior. The tragedy seems to be over.

But then he snaps. Suddenly doubting the justice of his actions, Orestes panics. He stares at the chorus and then, staring beyond them, shrieks that demons are coming to attack him (1048–56):

> **Orestes**: Ah, ah! I see these hideous women looking like Gorgons— clad in dark-grey tunics and thickly wreathed with serpents! I can't stay here.

> **Chorus**: Dearest of men to your father, what are these hallucinations (*doxai*) that are whirling about you? Hold firm, don't be afraid—you have won a great victory!

> **Orestes**: These afflictions are no hallucinations (*doxai*) I am having; these are plainly my mother's wrathful hounds!

> **Chorus**: Ah, the blood is still fresh on your hands; that, you see, is the cause of this confusion falling on your mind.[13]

The chorus protests that it cannot see these "demons" and assumes they are hallucinations, but it cannot convince Orestes that they are unreal. Seemingly in the grip of a psychotic break, the hero cries out (1061–2):

> **Orestes**: Lord Apollo, there are more and more of them! And they're dripping a loathsome fluid from their eyes! . . . You don't see these creatures, but I do! I'm being driven, driven away! I can't stay here!

With these words, Orestes flees the scene and the curtain falls.

The First Crucial Question: Are the Furies Real?

A "hallucination" is a self-reported imagining. Within the fiction of Aeschylus's play, are the demons Orestes says he sees real, or are they hallucinations? In *Eumenides*, the final play of Aeschylus' trilogy, the demons—more commonly called "Furies"—appear onstage as speaking characters. Because the action of *Eumenides* follows immediately on that of *Libation Bearers*, some classicists decide the Furies must be real in *Libation Bearers*, too. For example, in a recent popular student edition of *Libation Bearers*, Justina Gregory writes (2009, p. xxi):

> [T]here is no suggestion that the Furies are a delusion of Orestes' deranged mind. After all, the Furies will constitute the chorus in the next play; it would be perverse for Aeschylus to suggest that they are imaginary in one play and assign them major roles in the next. Rather, they are visible only to Orestes because their business is only with him.

Others disagree. In their view, it was in the interest of suspense, not perversity, that Aeschylus decided to tease his audience about the reality or unreality of Orestes' seemingly supernatural visions, and that suffices to explain why *Libation Bearers* ends precisely as it does: the ending is a cliffhanger. On this view, when the curtain rises in *Eumenides* to show that the Furies are really real, Aeschylus gave his audience a twist worthy of *The Sixth Sense*, the 1999 Hollywood film directed by M. Night Shyamalan. The surprise ending of that movie shocked audiences by suddenly revealing that within the fiction of the movie, supernatural elements really are real—and so retroactively, really *were* real all along.

Actually, this has been the preferred view since antiquity. The belief that the Furies appear as the consequence of Orestes undergoing a psychotic break—of him "going crazy"—is found at least as early as Sextus Empiricus (c. 160–210 AD), a physician and philosopher of Pyrrhonian Skepticism.[14] Glenn W. Most speaks for virtually all classicists today when he asserts, "The paradigmatic example of Greek tragic madness is Orestes," adding:

> Both Aeschylus [in *Libation Bearers*] and Euripides dedicate memorable and extended portrayals to the hero who, when he was relatively sane, committed the unspeakable crime of murdering his own mother, and later became a celebrated madman, pursued by the Erinyes

[= Furies] who sought to punish him for that deed. Are the Erinyes real divine instances that exist independently of Orestes' mental state, or are they projections of his quite understandable feelings of remorse and anguish for what he has done, or in some way a mixture of both? . . . [I]n Aeschylus, Orestes sees things that are simply not there in the physical dimension to which he assigns them. . . . As far as we can tell, it is the closing scene of Aeschylus' *Choephori* [*Libation Bearers*] that introduces crazed Orestes onto the stage of world literature; and it does so in such a memorable way that many of the later dramatic versions of his insanity are best seen as direct responses to Aeschylus' text.[15]

Most goes on to call the Furies visual hallucinations. Psychiatrist Nancy Andreasen shares this view: "In *The Oresteia*, Orestes is pursued by the Furies until he finally loses his reason and lapses into madness."[16]

In contemporary parlance, Most and Andreasen seem to believe that *Libation Bearers* ends with Orestes suffering from Post-Traumatic Stress Disorder, or PTSD. This interpretation alone makes sense of their assertions that Orestes killed his mother "when he was relatively sane," that Orestes "finally loses his reason and lapses into madness," and that "it is the *closing scene* of Aeschylus' *Choephori* [*Libation Bearers*] that introduces crazed Orestes onto the stage of world literature." An undated but ancient poem attributed to the lyric poet Anacreon (c. 582–c. 485 BC) takes the same view: "Alcmaeon and white-footed Orestes went crazy after they had killed their mothers."[17]

These statements show how the assumptions we bring to the closing scene of *Libation Bearers*—assumptions about the reality or unreality of the Furies—determine our interpretation of everything that precedes that scene. Before returning to this issue, let me now turn in a different direction and ask a simple question: Why exactly does Orestes kill his mother and her lover in *Libation Bearers*?

The Second Crucial Question: Has Apollo Really Been Speaking to Orestes?

Influential classicists assume or assert that Orestes kills his mother in obedience to a command of the oracular god Apollo. R. P. Winnington-Ingram declares, "Orestes is impelled towards matricide by Apollo."[18] For Helene P. Foley, "There can be no doubt that Orestes, in obedience to Apollo's command, has returned to Argos to carry out his revenge."[19] And in a recent introduction to the *Oresteia* meant for students, Simon Goldhill writes, "Orestes, however, is expressly instructed by Apollo to kill Clytemnestra. . . ." Goldhill adds that in *Libation Bearers*, "Orestes explains how Apollo is a direct controlling force for his action."[20]

Psychiatrists apparently share this reading of the play. Bennett Simon states:

> The form of the conflict for Orestes is stated quite explicitly in his speech beginning at line 269. Apollo has charged him to execute his mother and to avenge his father. If he fails to carry out the Delphic charge, he must suffer dire punishments. . . . I must reiterate that in Aeschylus these conflicts are located in the cosmos and in the society rather than in the individual. Orestes does not work through terrible inner conflicts in order to reach some sort of inner harmony.[21]

Having accepted this assumption uncritically and thereby authenticated it, classicists then allow it to color and inform their view of Greek religion. I submit that just as a forged painting, once accredited, allows all successive forgeries to be more easily accepted and thus gradually comes to distort our understanding of an artist's output, so too has our acceptance of Orestes' claims about Apollo at face value gradually come to distort our understanding of ancient Greek piety. For example, Ulrich von Wilamowitz-Moellendorf (1848–1931) is typically hailed as the greatest classical scholar of modern times, but he seems to have reversed premise and conclusion when he declared: "We all know that he [Apollo] made the avenging of blood an imperative duty upon men; Orestes slew his own mother at the god's command."[22] Worse, contemporary classicists go a step further and condone, characterize, or even endorse Orestes' killing of his mother as a "necessity," a necessity they attribute to the "divine command" of Apollo's oracle.[23]

This pat view of Apollo, Orestes, and the murder he commits is wrong. It resembles a pearl whose growth was stimulated by a single, minute grain of sand that found its way into the oyster's shell. What is the grain of sand? It is the assumption that in *Libation Bearers*, Orestes really has heard the real voice of Apollo—that is, god—commanding him to kill. Since this assumption has never been challenged, and since Szasz has shown us how best to unpack and assess such claims in contemporary times, I would like to examine the evidence for it in Aeschylus' play carefully.

Orestes' Claims About Apollo's Oracle

We first hear of Apollo's alleged injunction surprisingly late in the play. It comes as a startling revelation that Orestes casually makes in 269–74. After much ado, the hero tells his sister, Electra, and the chorus of Argive women (269–74):

> Loxias' [Apollo's] mighty oracle (*chrēsmos*) will *not* betray me. It's ordering (*keleuōn*) me to brave this peril, it's crying out (*exorthiazōn*) many things, and it is speaking plainly (*exaudomenos*) of catastrophes that will bring dire chill into my hot heart if I don't go after those guilty of my father's death "in the same manner"—saying (*legōn*), kill them in revenge.[24] He [Apollo] kept on saying (*ephaske*) I would pay for it myself with my own dear life, enduring many disagreeable sufferings, enfeebled by penalties that went beyond loss of property.

In Greek, an oracle (*chrēsmos*) can be a person, a place, or a voice of the god. As we can see, the emphasis here is firmly on Orestes' "hearing the voice" of Apollo. Where did he hear it, and when? Loxias is the cult title of Apollo at Delphi. By calling him that, Orestes might imply he heard the god's voice in an oracle at Delphi, but the play never hints at such a visit or even a motive that might have brought Orestes there. Quite the opposite; oddly, and unusually, Orestes' verbs imply that he is hearing Apollo's voice, or seems to be hearing it, right now, directly and in real time. That remains true throughout the play. Moreover, Orestes characterizes the divine voice as audible, commanding, menacing, and unambiguous. He portrays the orders it issues as irresistible.

It is also left unclear whether Orestes received this alleged oracle voluntarily or involuntarily. Did he—like Oedipus in Sophocles' *Oedipus Rex*—travel to Delphi on his own initiative and *ask* Apollo? Or did he somehow "hear" it—or is he even now hearing it, as he implies—against his will? These are crucial questions that Szasz taught us to ask, but the play never says.

Let me anticipate an objection that will also clarify my approach to assessing Orestes' claims. The first ten or twenty lines of *Libation Bearers* were lost in transmission from antiquity to today, and it is possible that Orestes mentioned a visit to Delphi in them.[25] Garvie raises this possibility, but only to dismiss it: "The only information which is missing [in the prologue], and which might have been given, concerns Orestes' mission from Apollo. . . . More probably there was no mention of this."[26] Either way, I would like to emphasize that the content of those missing verses makes no difference for my argument.

The reason is that it is Orestes himself who speaks the prologue, and he is merely a character in the play, not an omniscient narrator. If he says crazy things later in this play that we refuse to credit, therefore, there is no reason to accept statements he might have made in the prologue just because they appear in that prologue.

Although not usually so taken, therefore, I consider Orestes' words in 269–74 clear evidence that Orestes is (saying he is) experiencing "command delusions." In plain English, he says God's voice is ordering him to kill his mother. And he carries on for another thirty lines that grow increasingly detailed, bizarre, threatening, and mixed in their imagery, imagery that is not rooted in objective reality (275–96):

> He [Apollo] revealed (*piphaskōn*[27]) the effects of the wrath of hostile powers from under the earth against mortals, and spoke of these dreadful afflictions—leprous ulcers attacking the flesh, eating away its pristine appearance with savage jaws, and short white hairs arising on the disease site. He kept speaking (*ephōnei*) too of other assaults of Furies, generated by the blood of a father: the dark weapon of the powers below, arising from those of one's kin who have fallen and beg for justice, together with madness and empty nighttime terrors, derange him, harry him, and chase him from his city, physically humiliated by a metal collar. And men such as this, He said, are not permitted to have a share in the mixing bowl or in the pouring of a friendly libation; the father's unseen wrath keeps him away from altars; no one will receive him as a host or lodge with him as a guest, and finally he will die, devoid of all respect and devoid of all friends, cruelly shriveled in a death of total decay.

And yet just as Orestes seems to have convinced everyone that this supernaturalism is real and that within the play, Apollo at some point has given him special access to it, his tone suddenly lurches back to earth. He turns to his sister Electra and asks (297–311):

> Shouldn't I believe such an oracle as that? Even if I do not, the deed still has to be done. Many motives join together to point the same way: the command of the god, my great grief for my father, being deprived of my property weighs heavily on me . . . so that Argos's citizens, the most glorious people on earth, who overthrew Troy with resolute heart, should not remain, as they now are, subjected to a pair of women—for Aegisthus will soon know whether he really has a woman's heart or not!

What a revelation! Orestes has a litany of reasons for murdering his mother and her lover—some paranoid, some material, some

177

misogynistic. And Electra, the sister who has been deprived of the princess' life she expected to live, shares them fully.[28] This is made clear in a long scene in the middle of the play, a scene sufficiently famous that we find it illustrated on a south-Italian vase datable to c. 50 or 75 years after the debut of *Libation Bearers* in Athens (see figure 8.1).

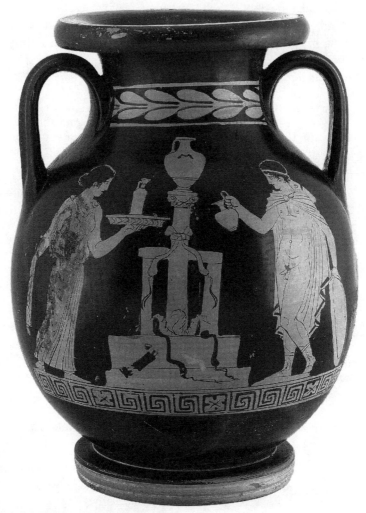

Figure 8.1. Red-figure pelike with Electra and Orestes at the tomb of their father Agamemnon. Apulia, Italy, attributed to the Tarporley Painter or his circle, c. 410–380 BC. Ceramic with painted decoration. Collection of the Herbert F. Johnson Museum of Art, Cornell University. Transfer from the History of Art Collection 74.74.007.

In the scene Orestes and Electra stand in front of their father's tomb and whip each other into an increasingly murderous frenzy of resentment and rage. They nurse and magnify their grievances, lionizing their dead father and demonizing their mother. Orestes prays to Zeus (pp. 255–258, 267–268):

> Look down on us!
> I and Electra, too, I tell you, children
> robbed of our father, both of us bound
> in exile from our house. . . .
> We seem in ruins now, I know. Up from nothing
> rear a house to greatness.

Abetted by the chorus, Orestes and Electra spiral into a fit of fury (379–90):

> **Orestes**: Zeus, Zeus, force up from the earth
> destruction, late but true to the mark,
> to the reckless heart, the killing hand—
> for parents of revenge revenge be done.
>
> **Chorus leader**: And the ripping cries of triumph mine
> to sing when the man is stabbed,
> the woman dies—
> why hide what's deep inside me,
> black wings beating, storming the spirit's prow—
> hurricane, slashing hatred!
>
> **Electra**: Both fists at once
> come down, come down—
> Zeus, crush their skulls! Kill! Kill!

Classicists read this scene and declare it a *kommos*, a "lamentation." I say it is an illustration of how a group of individuals, bereft of their father or father figure, transforms a gravesite into a martyr's shrine. Exaggerating the goodness of their dead father and the evil of their living mother, they fanaticize each other into believing that killing the one will avenge the other.

The scene is also an illustration of the kind of people who show up in the offices of analysts requesting psychoanalysis. As Szasz once quipped,

> Aided and abetted by corrupt analysts, patients who have nothing better to do with their lives often use the psychoanalytic situation to transform insignificant childhood hurts into private shrines at which

they worship unceasingly the enormity of the offenses committed against them.[29]

However we read Aeschylus' scene, the *"kommos"* is remarkable for the fact that no one in it mentions Apollo or his alleged oracle. The focus is entirely on the children's sense of financial destitution and dishonor.

"Command Hallucinations," Then and Now

What do such resentments and material motives mean for Orestes' "true" motive in killing his mother? If we assume Apollo's command is real, as critics do, we tie ourselves into knots. Deborah Roberts speaks for many in stating: "Orestes' vengeance is in some sense overmotivated; he is moved by the god's command, by his own grief for his father, and by his lost birthright (*Cho.* 299–304)."[30]

Yet even Orestes seems reluctant to believe his own alleged command hallucinations. He makes it clear he is play-acting. His words evoke the words of John Nash (1928–2015), the celebrity paranoid schizophrenic who won the Nobel Prize in Economic Sciences in 1994. "People are always selling the idea," remarked Nash, "that people with mental illness are suffering. . . . I think madness can be an escape. If things are not so good, you maybe want to imagine something better. In madness, I thought I was the most important person in the world."[31] This statement and point of view were not represented in *A Beautiful Mind*, the 2001 Hollywood film based on Nash's life. Szasz knew them, however, and he quoted them in *Words to the Wise* alongside a similar gem. Szasz drew attention to a man who complained of receiving messages from a loudspeaker in his classroom and becoming the object of a Mafia conspiracy. Evoking Aeschylus' Orestes, the man commented: "When you actually believe that, sometimes it's fun."[32]

There is a larger point to make about allegedly irresistible "command hallucinations." Szasz saw clearly that despite what we may tell ourselves, most of us do not really believe in this myth. He exposed the fallacy inherent in such claims succinctly (2004, pp. 60–61):

> I maintain that a person who believes he should kill someone—say, because he "hears voices" ordering him to do so—has only two legitimate choices: he can control himself and not kill another person, or he can kill himself.

Actually, we can go a step further. Although Szasz did not say so, the proof that we lack commitment to this mythic concept of uncontrollable "command delusions" can be seen in the fact that we are comfortable with murder as a metaphor, but not with rape as a metaphor. "My boss is killing me" can be said in polite company; whereas "My boss is raping me" cannot. Why? For the same reason that the insanity defense is tolerated for murder but not for rape. We realize that the sexual urge, unlike murder, really can be akin to an irresistible impulse; that is why custom, church, and state have always sought to limit its expression.

At any rate, Szasz's admonitions have fallen on deaf ears. The presence of "command delusions" is today regarded as a telltale symptom of (paranoid) schizophrenia. It is worth reminding ourselves of the others.

The Diagnostic Criteria of Paranoid Schizophrenia, and Some Recent Case Studies

Since the DSM-5 recently abolished the classical subtypes of schizophrenia, I will cite them from the DSM-IV:

> The essential feature of the paranoid type of schizophrenia is the presence of prominent delusions or auditory hallucinations. . . . Delusions are typically persecutory or grandiose, or both, but delusions with other themes (e.g., jealousy, religiosity, or somatization) may also occur. The delusions may be multiple, but are usually organized around a coherent theme. Associated features include anxiety, anger, aloofness, and argumentativeness. The individual may have a superior and patronizing manner and either a stilted, formal quality or extreme intensity in interpersonal interactions. . . . [T]he combination of persecutory and grandiose delusions with anger may predispose the individual to violence.

These criteria do not mention two corollaries that clinicians and the general public often take for granted: First, that schizophrenia tends to manifest in late adolescence (late teens to early twenties); second, that schizophrenic hallucinations are usually auditory, figured as "voices." The voices can express various ideas but usually fall into patterns. They may mock the individual who hears them or threaten him. As "command hallucinations," they may order him to harm himself or others. They may also suggest he enjoys exalted birth or that he has been chosen for a special, often divine, mission. Because psychiatrists arbitrarily exempt religious beliefs, Judaism, which meets the last two criteria, is not considered a symptom of schizophrenia. Yet until recently, about half of all schizophrenic delusions (or hallucinations) were religious in nature.[33]

These criteria describe Orestes in *Libation Bearers* exactly. He says he hears a voice commanding, threatening, and bullying him to harm others. He either has, or he thinks he has, been chosen for the special, divine mission of avenging his father. In fact, Orestes is strikingly similar to a number of young American men whose cases have appeared in recent newspaper reports. Herewith, some examples:

- The day after Christmas, 2013, Bobby Rankin of Deep River, Connecticut, picked up a fireplace poker and stabbed his mother to death. He cut open her torso with a hunting knife, then cleaned himself up and took his dog for a walk. He was 23 years old. Why did he do it? When police arrived Rankin told them, "I killed my mother because she is pretty much responsible for everything that has gone wrong in my life." According to his attorney, "Rankin thought his mother was an alien and that he had to hurt her because she was taking power from him." At trial, doctors testified that Rankin "is schizophrenic and has experienced severe psychosis." A panel of three judges found him not guilty by reason of insanity and committed him to a psychiatric hospital.[34]
- In 2006, eighteen-year-old Jeremy Hauck of Farmington City, Utah, shot his mother, slit her throat, and stuffed her body in a freezer. Police caught up with him in Montana, where he had fled in her car. "At the time he killed his mother," his attorney claimed, "he was hearing instructions from what he called 'The Source,' which he described as a 'data stream.' . . . [H]e thought a chip had been implanted [in his arm] that was giving him directions. 'The Source' told Hauck to kill his mother." Doctors diagnosed him with paranoid delusions and schizophrenia and a judge found him not guilty by reason of insanity.[35]
- On September 11, 2015, forty-year-old Wisconsin man Matthew J. Skalitzky beheaded his mother with a four-foot-long sword at the condo that she and her husband owned and had allowed him to live in. A roommate heard the mother screaming "No, no, no." Going upstairs he found Skalitzky holding the sword and covered in blood. Skalitzky acknowledged killing her but told the police "she's not my real mother." A psychiatrist has found him incompetent to stand trial, and he is currently being held in a mental health facility. Press reports speculate that he is schizophrenic.[36]

Sadly, these examples could be easily multiplied, and it is not hard to spot a pattern among them.[37] It is that unmistakable combination of arrogance, dependence, claims of hearing voices, and violence against their relatives that we call schizophrenia.

What do these accounts teach us? Today, when a young man on the cusp of manhood says he hears voices and murders his mother, we declare him mentally ill rather than guilty or evil. We diagnose him as a (paranoid) schizophrenic and confine him in a mental institution. In ancient Greece, when a young man on the cusp of manhood says he hears voices and murders his mother, we credit his claims that God told him to do it and pathologize the voice of his conscience—the "Furies" that he says have arisen to torment him—as PTSD.

Throughout his career, Szasz traced the origin of man's displacement of responsibility onto "mental illness" sprung from alleged brain diseases only to the Enlightenment.[38] On that score, he must be corrected. I would now like to demonstrate that the claims characteristic of schizophrenia were well known in Europe before the advent of Christianity, and that even two thousand years ago such claims and concerns were sometimes regarded as a matter of medicine.

Hearing Voices, Then and Now; The Evidence of Plautus' *The Menaechmus Brothers*

Did people in ancient Greece and Rome claim to hear schizophrenic "voices"? Yes. The proof is a stage comedy titled *The Menaechmus Brothers* by the Roman playwright Plautus (254–184 BC), a comedy that has not been discussed in connection with Aeschylus' *Libation Bearers* before. At its climax (831–88), the play's protagonist pretends to hear the voice of Apollo commanding him to kill his wife and father-in-law.

The Menaechmus Brothers is a comedy of mistaken identity. It is dated to c. 200 BCE but is based on a lost Greek comedy of c. 350 BC or earlier. Unlike Aeschylus' *Libation Bearers*, however, which is set in a remote and legendary past, Plautus' play is set in the real world of its time and shows us a lightly distorted mirror of daily life in Hellenistic Greece. As I have contended elsewhere, the play's central concern is the nature of insanity.[39]

Late in the play a young stranger in the Greek city of Epidamnus, named Menaechmus, suddenly finds himself in fear of the law (831–75). The only escape he can think of is to feign "insanity" (*insania*) in hopes of scaring people away. What does he do? He pretends to hear Apollo's voice ordering him to kill his wife and father-in-law. The scene in question begins with Menaechmus turning to the audience, breaking the dramatic illusion, and asking us a rhetorical question (831–2):

> Since they're claiming I'm insane (*insanire*), what better could I do than pretend I *am* insane (*insanire*), and scare them off of me?

And all of a sudden—he pretends—Apollo's voice is commanding him to attack his wife. Feigning a psychotic break he cries out:

> There! Apollo from his oracle is commanding me
> to take some hotly blazing torches, set this woman's eyes on fire!
> (840–1)

> (*to Apollo*) Do not spare my fists in punching her face,
> unless she hurries out of sight and quickly goes to hell?
> Yes, Apollo, I will obey your command. (pp. 848–850)

Then he turns his attention to her father, and threatens him with increasing violence:

> (*to Apollo*) What's my orders? Beat the fellow limb from limb and bone from bone?
> Use the very stick he carries for the job? . . .
> I will obey your command: take a double axe and this old fogey,
> chop his innards into little pieces, till I reach the bone? (855–6, 858–9)

> Apollo! You command so much. Now you're ordering me to hitch up horses,
> wild, ferocious horses, and then mount up in my chariot,
> then to trample on this lion—creaking, stinking, toothless lion?
> (*feigning the motions*) And already I'm in the chariot, already got the reins, I've already got the whip . . . ! (862–5)

> Once again, Apollo, yea,
> you're ordering me to charge and kill the man that's standing here.
> (869–70)

In my view, these alleged command hallucinations constitute proof positive that ancient theater audiences were familiar with the kind of individuals who claim God is telling them to commit violence, and that those audiences were as unwilling as people today are to credit those claims as authentic divine revelation. The scene also demonstrates that ancient audiences were prepared to attribute these bizarre claims to brain disease and seek chemical cures for them. As the scene closes, Menaechmus's violence so disturbs the father-in-law that in 872–4 he blurts out: "Good grief! He's *ill*—and how!" In so doing, the father-in-law explicitly connects "insanity" with "illness" (*morbus*). Alarmed and concerned, he runs off to get a psychiatrist (*medicus*). And as I have discussed elsewhere, he returns with a doctor of Hippocratic (scientific) medicine, who promptly prescribes a course of forcible drugging and confinement as treatment.[40]

Anticipating an Objection

In returning to *Libation Bearers*, I would like to anticipate a potential misunderstanding. In denying the validity of Orestes' claims about Apollo, it is not necessary to assert—and I am not asserting, since it is probably untrue—that Aeschylus was an atheist. Catholic priests and Jewish rabbis routinely summon a psychiatrist when a parishioner tells them God is urging him to hurt himself or someone else, and summoning a psychiatrist does nothing to diminish their belief in the existence or intervention of God. In fact, as Szasz recognized, such cases seem to achieve the opposite effect. Because (as a matter of theological principle) religious leaders refuse to believe God would issue so evil an order, these cases wind up reaffirming both their belief in God's inherent goodness *and* their commitment to the psychiatric interpretation of problems in living. That remarkable outcome tells us a great deal about the human condition.

An example will illustrate this point. In October 2012, twenty-year-old Matt Stick of Tulsa, Oklahoma, stabbed his mother to death on her front porch. The two had been watching an apocalyptic-themed television show:

> "[A] character's weapon triggered a hunch that evil was lurking. The 20-year-old [Matt Stick] jumped into action, his brain working on instinct to save his mother, Veronica Stick, from the demons. After stabbing her with a knife he thought was blessed by God, he believed that her gasps indicated a monster leaving. . . .

> Covered in blood, he headed to his job at All Souls Unitarian Church, eventually abandoning his car in a Brookside neighborhood and walking to the church. He was disoriented but not fleeing.

> "I thought I was doing what God wanted me to do," Stick said. "I thought I was a spiritual warrior or demon hunter. . . . [In high school] he started hearing people speak in unknown languages. "I heard strange voices, and thought I was experiencing something religious or spiritual," he said. "Then I started experiencing very, very strange things. I thought my dog was communicating with me telepathically. I knew that was weird."

> "The 'voice' I heard wasn't so much auditory but more like a sixth sense," Stick said. "I could sense or smell evil, and I felt I had to

do something about it. I had to act quickly. That is what led to my mother's death." . . .

Following his arrest, doctors diagnosed him with bipolar disorder with paranoid delusions. He was found not guilty of stabbing his mother to death on the grounds of insanity.[41]

Matt Stick's father, Michael Stick, is a Baptist minister. He maintains a Facebook page in which he declares, "My son is my life. . . . If you believe in prayer, I ask that you pray for God's presence, comfort, peace, and patience in his life."[42]

The evil that Michael Stick's son did to his mother did nothing to shake the father's faith in God. I am suggesting that Aeschylus held a similar view of Apollo in *Libation Bearers*—and that his audience readily agreed with him.

Summing Up

The canonical interpretation of *Libation Bearers* gets it exactly backward. Orestes does not go crazy at the end of the play. It would be more correct to say that he is already crazy at the start of the play. Yet what exactly does that mean?

In dramatizing the legend of Orestes, Aeschylus faced a peculiar challenge. He inherited a tradition in which Orestes killed his mother on the order of Apollo. That story is easier told than shown. The challenge to the playwright was to make that narrative scenario seem plausible as a stage drama. His solution, and stroke of genius, was to portray Orestes as the type of man that we call a paranoid schizophrenic. It is only at the close of the play, when he wants to transition to *Eumenides*, the sequel play, that he begins to prepare us for the possibility that Apollo's intervention was real all along. Before then, the alleged "oracle" is constantly characterized as either Apollo's direct and actual "voice" that Orestes thinks he is hearing, as in Plautus' *The Menaechmus Brothers*, or as an archetypal "influencing machine," no different from the claims heard in our time about messages beamed through telegraphs, loudspeakers, dental fillings, televisions, the internet, and so on.

This assumption reduces Orestes' overdetermined motive for killing his mother—"the command of the god, my great grief for my father, being deprived of my property"—to a typical motive, the kind we read about every week. It also solves a longstanding mystery about *Libation Bearers*. In 1959 Marie Delcourt (1891–1979), professor of classical philology at the University of Liege and an acknowledged expert on Greek religion, studied the claims made about Apollo's oracle in the play and reached two conclusions: First, that "no known oracle offers the slightest resemblance to the one in *Libation Bearers*," and second, that "the oracle in *Libation Bearers* does not include any doctrine that can be considered Delphic."[43] She was unable to find any other oracles in Greek life or literature that commanded one person to kill another. Yet having gazed into the abyss, she averted her eyes in a way that brings to mind a dictum that Szasz was fond of quoting. "If you miss the first buttonhole," remarked Goethe, "you will not succeed in buttoning up your coat."[44] Delcourt's findings did nothing to change the interpretation of the play.

Orestes is not a divinely appointed avenger. He is simply the kind of young man that calls himself one. He is pompous and grandiose; in the play's first scene he sees himself as literally the answer to his sister's prayers (212–5) and, in a later scene, as the literal fulfillment of his mother's nightmare (528–37). His companion, Pylades, is not a representative of Apollo; he is simply a loyal follower who has converted to the cause of Orestes, a follower who believes his master's self-serving lies even more sincerely than the master does. That explains why at the climax of the play, when Orestes momentarily doubts himself, Pylades eggs him on and reassures him of the justice of their mission (886–9). Hence, no wonder the "furies" rise up to torment Orestes: they are not supernatural agents "driving" him crazy, much less "hallucinations" symptomatic of a brain disease. They are simply an example of what the late psychologist Theodore Sarbin (1911–2005) called a self-disavowed imagining.[45]

Nevertheless, I predict my interpretation of *Libation Bearers* will fail. Classicists will dismiss it because psychiatrists tell them schizophrenia is a brain disease of recent origin. Psychiatrists will dismiss it because classicists tell them Orestes really does, within his own cultural context, hear the voice of God. Let me therefore enter a final plea.

Most people today continue to credit the concept of "hearing voices"—selectively credit it, of course, since outside of the Old Testament, no one believes the claim that God really commands people to harm one other. That is one pillar on which the medical disease concept of schizophrenia rests. Rejecting that belief suggests that Szasz was correct when he observed, "If you talk to God, you are praying. If God talks to you, you have schizophrenia."[46] Yet if we refuse to credit those claims, then what are delusions of persecution? According to Szasz, the answer is simple. It is existential:

> Jones is an extra on the stage of life. He wants to be a star. He cannot become a star by making a fortune on the stock market or winning a Nobel Prize. Instead, he claims that the FBI or the Communists are watching his every move, tapping his phone, sending him coded messages. They would not be doing this if he were not a very important person.

> A paranoid delusion is a problem to the so-called patient's family and friends. For the "patient," it is a solution for the problem of the meaning(lessness) of life.[47]

The conclusion is clear. Those who favor the recency hypothesis of schizophrenia say it is like the AIDS epidemic. Aeschylus' *Libation Bearers* suggests a more appropriate comparison is obesity, another skyrocketing "epidemic" (and mental illness *in statu nascendi*) whose "causes" are social and personal rather than infectious or cellular. It suggests the *causes of* schizophrenia are really *reasons for* schizophrenia. I thus arrive at an interpretation of (paranoid) schizophrenia squarely in line with that propounded by Szasz:

> The paranoid schizophrenic is the person who craves recognition too eagerly and too impatiently: He is too ambitious, too energetic, too conceited; he cannot wait, work, and create the context in which his worth will be recognized by others.

> By the time he reaches his late teens or early twenties, he feels the time has come for people to recognize him as the superior person he is. He becomes arrogant and haughty, overplays his hand, and plummets to earth, a human wreck. His craving for attention unfulfilled, he imagines that people are watching him, spying on him, harassing him: he is, once again, a *wunderkind*, the center of attention.

> In short, paranoid schizophrenia is a kind of premature existential ejaculation.[48]

Characteristically, Szasz's observation is both witty and profound. To judge from Aeschylus' *Libation Bearers*, it is also correct.

* * *

Every now and then an extraordinary thinker is born, a thinker who sees through the mass delusions of his time and has the courage, or the hardihood, to say so. Thomas Szasz was one. Like the philosophers Epicurus or Schopenhauer, he took it for granted that God is a fiction; that human affairs are ruled by custom and metaphor rather than reason or clarity; and that human beings are as apt to lie to themselves as we are to one another. Like them, he allowed his thoughts to roam fearlessly outward to their natural endpoints and to see things as they actually are.

The classicist asked to assess the legacy of Thomas Szasz finds precedents everywhere he looks. In *The Myth of Mental Illness* Szasz is Prometheus, defying authority in hopes of helping mankind. In his tenure battle early in his career he is Daedalus, surviving the odds by his ingenuity but unable to save the younger followers who sided with him and crashed to earth. And in *The Medicalization of Everyday Life* he is Euhemerus, the spoilsport who finds simpler, less sensational explanations to the great myths that bring order to our lives. Probably because he learned English only late and as the object of deliberate study, he understood that the correct use of language is the key to distinguishing phenomena from attributes, literal speech from metaphor, and myth from reality.

Someday Szasz will be hailed as a pillar of Western civilization, but that day is still far off. The problem with a mass delusion is that by definition, only the heretics know when we are living through one. The rest of us can't tell. In seventeenth century Europe, everyone knew they had an immortal soul and that witches could harm it. Today, it seems, everyone knows that the soul is just the brain and that medical doctors can heal it. Szasz realized that assumption was false and devoted his life to saying so. The great but simple truth that he derived from it, and from which all his subsequent ideas flow, is that faith in medicine is still faith, not medicine.

Notes

1. *De Rerum Natura* 1.62–71; tr. Bailey (1910), modified.
2. Orwell (1946).
3. Schopenhauer (1862) vol. 2, 227: ". . . sie sind ein Schandfleck der ganzen Menschheit."
4. Szasz (1988).
5. Wiseman (1967), which is no longer banned, offers one glimpse inside a mental hospital.
6. Andreasen (1999).
7. NIMH (2015).
8. Torrey (2011).
9. Gottesmann (1991); Noll (2007, pp. xi–xiii); Jablensky et al. (2011, p. 195).

10. Evans et al. (2003).
11. Centers for Disease Control and Prevention (2012).
12. In English *Libation Bearers* is the standard title, but the play is also often referred to by its Greek title *Choephori* or *Choephoroe*.
13. In this paper I usually cite *Libation Bearers* in the translation of Sommerstein (2009), occasionally modified, though elsewhere I have preferred that of Fagles (1984).
14. *Against Logicians* 1.170, 244, 249; 2.63, 67, cited in Most (2013, p. 403).
15. Most (2013, pp. 398–399), with my insertions in brackets.
16. Andreasen (2011, p. 4).
17. Anacreontea 9.
18. Winnington-Ingraham (1983, p. 136).
19. Foley (2001, p. 33).
20. Goldhill (2004, pp. 53 and 68).
21. Simon (1978, pp. 103 and 108).
22. Wilamowitz (1908, p. 39).
23. Thus Roberts (1984, p. 39).
24. In 270ff. Sommerstein translates these present participles with past tense verbs. I retain the present tense.
25. Garvie (1986, p. 47) estimates fewer than ten lines are missing; Bowen (1991, p. 27) thinks "10 or 20."
26. Garvie (1986, p. 47).
27. This verb can mean either to say or to show. It more commonly means to say.
28. See lines 130–137.
29. Szasz (2004, pp. 175–176).
30. Roberts (1984, p. 29).
31. Nash (2002).
32. Szasz (2004, pp. 198, 199).
33. Krzystanek et al. (2012).
34. Owens (2015); Griffin (2015).
35. Winslow (2013).
36. Winfrey (2016).
37. Recent examples include Gates (2015); Schoenfeld (2016); and Johnson (2007) and Doege (2007).
38. Szasz (2011).
39. Fontaine (2013).
40. Fontaine (2013).
41. Graham (2015).
42. Stick (2014).
43. Delcourt (1959, pp. 107 and 109): "I. Aucun oracle connu n'offre la moindre ressemblance avec celui des Choéphores. . . . II. L'oracle des Choéphores n'inclut aucune doctrine qui puisse être considérée comme delphique."
44. Szasz (2011, p. 186).
45. Sarbin (1990).
46. Szasz (2004, p. 196).
47. Szasz (2004, p. 199).
48. Szasz (2004, p. 137).

References

Andreasen, N. (1999, February 25). Editorial: Understanding the causes of schizophrenia. *New England Journal of Medicine, 340,* 645–647.

Andreasen, N. (2011). Concept of schizophrenia: Past, present, and future. In D. R. Weinberger & P. J. Harrison (Eds.), *Schizophrenia* (3rd ed.). Oxford: Wiley-Blackwell.

Bailey, C. (Trans.). (1910). *Titus Lucretius Carus: On the nature of things.* Oxford: Clarendon Press.

Bowen, A. A. (Ed.). (1991). *Aeschylus: Choephori.* Bristol: Classical Press.

Centers for Disease Control and Prevention. (2012). Monitoring selected national HIV prevention and care objectives by using HIV surveillance data—United States and 6 U.S. dependent areas. *2010 Surveillance Supplemental Report, 17*(3, Pt. A). Retrieved on February 6, 2015, from http://www.cdc.gov/hiv/pdf

Delcourt, M. (1959). *Oreste et Alcméon. Étude sur la projection légendaire du matricide en Grèce.* Paris: Éd. Belles-Lettres.

Doege, D. (2007, November 10). Ax killer's fate up to judge. *Milwaukee-Wisconsin Journal Sentinel.* Retrieved February 6, 2015, from http://www.jsonline.com/news/waukesha/29283699.html

Evans, K., McGrath, J., & Milns, R. (2003). Searching for schizophrenia in ancient Greek and Roman literature: A systematic review. *Acta Psychiatrica Scandinavica, 107*(5), 323–330. Retrieved February 6, 2015, from http://www.ncbi.nlm.nih.gov/pubmed/12752027

Fagles, R. (Trans.). *Aeschylus: The Oresteia: Agamemnon; The libation bearers; The Eumenides.* New York: Barnes & Noble.

Fontaine, M. (2013). On being sane in an insane place—The laboratory of plautus' epidamnus. *Current Psychology, 32,* 348–365.

Garvie, A. F. (Ed.). (1986). *Aeschylus: Choephori.* Oxford: Oxford University Press.

Gates, J. E. (2015, July 31). Mentally ill man who kills mother may get inheritance. *The Clarion-Ledger.* Web. Retrieved February 6, 2015, from http://www.clarionledger.com/story/news/2015/07/31/mentally-ill-man-who-kills-mother-may-get-inheritance/30959669/

Goldhill, S. (2004). *Aeschylus: The Oresteia. Landmarks of world literature* (2nd ed.). Cambridge: Cambridge University Press.

Gottesmann, I. I. (1991). *Schizophrenia genesis: The origins of madness.* New York: W. H. Freeman and Company.

Graham, G. (2015, June 10). Legally insane: A son talks about his actions, feelings about his mother's death. *Tulsa World.* Retrieved February 6, 2015, from http://www.tulsaworld.com/news/ginniegraham/legally-insane-a-son-talks-about-his-actions-feelings-about/article_1f81a082-2304-51b1-84b5-311697444baa.html

Gregory, J. (2009). Introduction. In Aeschylus, Peter Meineck, C. A. E. Luschnig, Paul Woodruff, Euripides, and Sophocles (Eds.), *The Electra plays.* Indianapolis, IN: Hackett.

Griffin, A. (2015, August 20). Deep river man committed for 60 years in mother's killing. *Hartford Courant.* Web. Retrieved February 6, 2015, from

http://www.courant.com/news/connecticut/hc-robert-rankin-psychiatric
-commitment-0821-20150820-story.html

Jablensky, A., Kirkbride, J. B., & Jones, P. B. (2011). Schizophrenia: The epidemi-
ological horizon. In D. R. Weinberger & P. J. Harrison (Eds.), *Schizophrenia*
(3rd ed.). Oxford: Wiley-Blackwell.

Johnson, M. (2007, November 30). Man gets life in ax murder. JSOnline.
Retrieved February 6, 2015, from http://www.freerepublic.com/focus
/news/1933654/posts

Krzystanek, M., Krysta, K., Klasik, A., & Krupka-Matuszczyk, I. (2012).
Religious content of hallucinations in paranoid schizophrenia. *Psychiatria
Danubina, 24*(Suppl 1), 65–69. Retrieved February 6, 2015, from http://
www.ncbi.nlm.nih.gov/pubmed/22945191

Most, G. W. (2013). The madness of tragedy. In W. V. Harris (Ed.), *Mental
disorders in the classical world* (pp. 395–410). Leiden, MA and Boston,
MA: Brill.

Nash, J. (2002). *A brilliant madness*. PBS television program. Retrieved
February 6, 2015, from www.pbs.org/wgbh/amex/nash/filmmore/pt.html

NIMH (National Institute of Mental Health) website. Schizophrenia.
Retrieved February 6, 2015, from http://www.nimh.nih.gov/health/topics
/schizophrenia/index.shtml

Noll, R. (2007). Madness, psychosis, schizophrenia: A brief history. In R. Noll
(Ed.), *The encyclopedia of schizophrenia and other psychotic disorders* (3rd
ed., pp. ix–xx). New York: Facts on File.

Ortiz, K. (2014, July 24). Police: Orange man, 22, accused of killing
mother, 58. *New Haven Register News*. Retrieved February 6, 2015,
from http://www.nhregister.com/general-news/20140724/police
-orange-man-22-accused-of-killing-mother-58

Orwell, G. In front of your nose (1946). Retrieved February 6, 2015, from
http://orwell.ru/library/articles/nose/english/e_nose

Owens, D. (2015, June 5). Deep river man who killed mother found not guilty
by reason of insanity. *Hartford Courant*. Web. Retrieved February 6, 2015,
from http://www.courant.com/breaking-news/hc-middletown-deep-river
-murder-0606-20150605-story.html

Roberts, D. H. (1984). *Apollo and his oracle in the oresteia*. Goettingen:
Vandenhoeck & Ruprecht.

Sarbin, T. R. (1990). Toward the obsolescence of the schizophrenia hypothesis.
The Journal of Mind and Behavior, 11, 259–284.

Schoenfeld, S. (2016, January 20). Man from Orange sentenced to 60 years in
psychiatric hospital for killing mother. *Fox61.com*. Retrieved February 6,
2015, from http://fox61.com/2016/01/20/man-from-orange-sentenced-to
-60-years-in-psychiatric-hospital-for-killing-mother/

Schopenhauer, A. (1862). *Parerga und paralipomena: Kleine philosophische
schriften* (2nd ed.), edited by Julius Frauenstaedt. Berlin: Verlagsort.

Shay, J. (2010). *Achilles in Vietnam: Combat trauma and the undoing of character*. New York: Simon and Schuster.

Simon, B. (1978). *Mind and madness in Ancient Greece. The classical roots of
modern psychiatry*. Ithaca, NY: Cornell University Press.

Sommerstein, A. (Ed. and Trans.). (2009). *Aeschylus II: Oresteia (Agamemnon; Libation-Bearers; Eumenides)*. Boston, MA: Harvard University Press (Loeb edition).

Stick, M. (2014, March 16). Retrieved February 6, 2015, from https://www.facebook.com/michael.stick.94/posts/615482578518512

Szasz, T. S. (1988). [1976]. *Schizophrenia: The sacred symbol of psychiatry.* Syracuse: Syracuse University Press.

Szasz, T. (1995). Idleness and lawlessness in the therapeutic state, *Society, May/June*, 30–35.

Szasz, T. (2004). *Words to the wise: A medical-philosophical dictionary.* New Brunswick: Transaction.

Szasz, T. (2011). *Coercion as cure: A critical history of psychiatry.* New Brunswick: Transaction.

Torrey, E. F. (2011). Schizophrenia as a brain disease: Studies of individuals who have never been treated—Backgrounder. Retrieved February 6, 2015, from http://www.treatmentadvocacycenter.org/resources/briefing-papers-and-fact-sheets/159/466

Weinberger, D. R., & Harrison, P. J. (Eds.). (2011). *Schizophrenia* (3rd ed.) Oxford: Wiley-Blackwell.

Wilamowitz-Moellendorff, U. von. (1908). *Greek historical writing, and Apollo: Two lectures delivered before the University of Oxford June 3 and 4, 1908.* Translated by Gilbert Murray. Oxford: Clarendon Press.

Winfrey, L. (2016, February 4). Update: Sun Prairie man in court for competency hearing. *NBC15.com.* Retrieved February 6, 2015, from www.nbc15.com/home/headlines/BREAKING--Domestic-dispute-situation-in-Sun-Prairie-326770121.html

Winnington-Ingram, R. P. (1983). *Studies in Aeschylus.* Cambridge: Cambridge University Press.

Winslow, B. (2013, March 4). Man who killed mom, stuffed her body in a freezer not guilty by reason of insanity. *Fox13now.com.* Retrieved February 6, 2015, from http://fox13now.com/2013/03/04/man-who-killed-mom-stuffed-her-body-in-a-freezer-not-guilty-by-reason-of-insanity/

Wiseman, F. (1967). *Titicut follies.* Cambridge, MA: Production Zipporah Films.

Part IV

Afterthoughts

9

The Seeds Tom Planted

Jeffrey A. Schaler

Although we may not know it, we have, in our day, witnessed the birth of the Therapeutic State. This is perhaps the major implication of psychiatry as an institution of social control.
—*Thomas Szasz, 1963*

Congress shall make no law respecting an establishment of medicine, or prohibiting the free exercise thereof...
—*Thomas S. Szasz, 1970*

Where does this leave us?

After I gave invited Grand Rounds to the psychiatry department at Upstate Medical University in Syracuse, January 2015, Mantosh Dewan, MD, the former chair of that department while Thomas Szasz was alive, came running up and asked, "Jeff, when do you think Tom's ideas will take hold, that is, finally be accepted?" I was kicking off a year of monthly Grand Round invitational talks to celebrate and remark on the importance of Thomas Szasz having worked there for over sixty years, the implications and significance of his life in general. I said I thought Tom was at least one hundred years ahead of his time. Who knows how long it will take? I am not optimistic.

Clearly, Tom was also a genius, and like many geniuses ahead of him, he is still scorned as a renegade, a heretic. He grasped incredibly erudite issues of philosophy, medicine, science, law, and psychology with grace and ease, the way Bach, Mozart and Beethoven may have grabbed inaudible melodies from some invisible metaphysical field, and translated them into a language that everyman could not only understand but also delight in. More than once someone remarked at his deft use of the English language. I remember how he responded, almost apologetically, "well, English is my second language."

Tom invited me, and I in turn others, (including my dear friend Bruce K. Alexander, an important contributor to this volume) to join him at a special conference of First Nations People in Edmonton, Alberta, November 1995. (Before I met Tom I spent fourteen years studying and practicing the martial arts, specifically Korean Kendo and Iaido—Myosim style, through which I had achieved my third degree black belt, no small accomplishment.) When I introduced Tom, as he often requested, I included the following story from *Zen and Japanese Culture* by D.T. Suzuki, as my own thinking and behavior remains influenced by the unwritten code of the Samurai, the Bushido (http://www.schaler.net/albertaintro.html):

> As far as the edge of the blade is concerned, Masamune, a master swordsmith of the Kamakura era in Japan, may not exceed Muramasa, one of his ablest disciples, but Masamune is said to have something morally inspiring that comes from his personality: When someone was trying to test the sharpness of a Muramasa, he placed it in a current of water and watched how it acted against the dead leaves flowing down stream. He saw that every leaf that met the blade was cut in twain. He then placed a Masamune, and he was surprised to find that the leaves avoided the blade. (Suzuki, 1973)

> To me, Thomas Szasz is Masamune.

Tom's humor was infectious and even his staunchest adversaries could not resist a bow. Too many critics interpreted what he wrote about in ways that were just *non sequiturs*. While many libertarians acknowledge him as a hero, when it comes to understanding what he meant by the myth of mental illness, they told me on numerous occasions that his ideas about mental illness were crazy, often without addressing them substantively. This was more than a little disconcerting to those of us who consider ourselves classical liberals, that is, libertarians, understanding and comprehending the meaning of his work. Tom and I concluded that too many libertarians were concerned only with economics at the expense of morality, ethics, human dignity, freedom, and responsibility.

I believe there are several reasons why people, especially psychiatrists and those in the mental health professions, resist Tom's ideas so, to the point of not even reading primary sources of Szasz. Tom's writings have undermined and falsified the claim that mental illness exists, that behavior can be a disease. Many people are invested in the myth of mental illness. They make money off the myth. They enjoy power over others off the myth. And families and friends who do not understand why loved ones behave in such disturbing ways are given a comforting cause and theory regarding treatment. They are also off the hook in terms of their own guilt. (As we all know, parents can drive their children crazy, and vice versa.) Psychiatrists and mental health professionals could engage in contractual psychotherapy if they wanted to do so. They obviously fear that they won't be able to support themselves and their families if they choose to go that route. Many patients may be unwilling to spend the money necessary for psychotherapy, if the cost of psychotherapy was not reimbursed by health insurance companies. Health insurance companies depend on the idea that mental illness is a treatable disease. It is the *investment* in the myth that we must consider.

While researchers are busy getting funded to find a physiological cause for schizophrenia, bipolar disease, depression, anxiety-based disorders, and so on, few people stop to realize there can never be a discrete variable called "mental illness." Tom and I concurred on this point privately on numerous occasions. The variable "schizophrenia" is impossible to define or quantify in a statistically meaningful way. This is true for any and all of the behaviors listed in the *Diagnostic and Statistical Manual of Mental Disorders, Volume* 5 (American Psychiatric Association, 2016; Schaler et al., 2012). The way schizophrenia is operationally defined includes, must include, hallucinations, hallucinations of any of the senses. These include auditory, visual, and tactile self-reported imaginings. To elaborate briefly on one of Tom's most popular aphorisms,

> *If you talk to God, you are praying;*
> *If God talks to you, you have schizophrenia.* (Szasz, 1973)

As I have discussed elsewhere, there are socially acceptable hallucinations or self-reported imaginings, for example, religious hallucinations, and socially unacceptable hallucinations, for example those diagnosed as schizophrenia, psychosis, and so on. There is no physical distinction between the two, and there never will be, because the distinction is a value judgment based on social and cultural mores. This, I believe, is extremely important. For one, if a physical lesion were discovered that could predict the occurrence of mental illness with an accuracy beyond that expected by chance, then a brain disease of biological, histological, or genetic origin would have been discovered, NOT a mental illness. The phenomenon would immediately belong to the realm of physical scientists, not metaphysical or political scientists—nosologists and pathologists, especially neurologists. As it stands, mental illnesses are not included in standard textbooks on pathology because they do not meet the nosological criteria for classification.

The fact that the reliability of the different categories of mental illness in the DSM has increased over the years, says nothing about the validity of those categories and diagnoses. Remember, there is no such thing as schizophrenia, or mental illness. Don't be fooled by enthymemes.

Mental illness refers to behaviors exhibited by people who disturb others. Behaviors are heterogeneous. Like snowflakes, no two are identical. Thus one could not generalize a finding in one to others with any degree of accuracy similar to that established with real diseases. When genetic researchers discover a gene accounting for a very specific type of breast cancer, the cancer variable is discrete, clearly defined. Compare that to a behavior called "schizophrenia" and we are faced with the obvious.

Years ago I asked a friend of mine about this, someone who had spent his career as a geneticist at the National Institutes of Health in Bethesda, Maryland. He said the following to me, when I asked him what he thought about claims that an allele or gene for alcoholism had been discovered: "Jeffrey, a gene for alcoholism or mental illness is absurd thinking from a genetic point of view. Even when we think we have found a specific allele for a specific and unique type of kidney disease, we are extremely reluctant to say a causal relationship exists. There are too many factors we may have missed." As my doctoral advisor, Robert Huebner, at the University of Maryland College Park never ceased to remind me, "there are plausible alternative explanatory hypotheses that may not have been accounted for in claims regarding a correlation." Statistical implications and conclusions demand, as anyone with a PhD has grown to learn, skepticism and caution first.

So why are researchers continually searching for a relationship that simply cannot exist? Because people abhor a vacuum when it comes to understanding troubling events and activities. They want to be able to say that "a" causes "b" because it gives a sense of existential comfort and security as well as the reassurance that the troubling phenomena may eventually be controlled and destroyed. Saying "I don't know" is taboo. Plus, searching for an impossible relationship, explained and justified using scientific rhetoric, assures the researchers of a job and income for years to come. When researchers announced that an allele for alcoholism had been discovered, the news was on all the major television networks and headlined major newspapers. Six months later researchers at NIH attempting to replicate the findings found the genetic allele not only was not significant in predicting alcoholism, it was more prevalent in nonalcoholics. I remember asking my students why the first study received so much attention, while the second study, a far more controlled study, ended up buried eight pages after the front page, and was but a passing small story. "Because that is not what the American people want to hear," said one student loudly. I could not have put it better (Schaler, 1990).

Most psychiatrists believe rather strongly in the validity of mental illness as they leave medical school and psychiatric residences. They spend a tremendous amount of money and time in school. Working with patients, diagnosing and prescribing medications, and making decisions regarding whether to incarcerate or hospitalize innocent or guilty persons weighs heavily on their minds. The courts and branches of state and federal government imbue them with considerable authority and expertise. And their patients and the lay public frequently regard them with considerable disdain and skepticism ("you must be crazy to see a psychiatrist!"). Moreover, they are very difficult to understand because they use pseudo-medical terminology.

"Real" physicians frequently differ significantly from psychiatrists. Many physicians refer to psychiatrists as fake doctors prescribing for "P" deficiency, as in Prozac deficiency. Also, real physicians take and abide by an oath not to treat someone without his consent. They also do not make determinations regarding criminal liability.

The two activities society appears most loath to give up are involuntary commitment and the insanity defense, regardless of how much these practices conflict with the U.S. Constitution. These are the Siamese twins of mental illness—institutional psychiatry and the insanity defense—that Tom always came back to, year after year. As Tom repeated, mind does not exist in a tangible, literal way, brain and mind are different, behavior cannot be a disease, whether a physiological correlate or cause for mental illness will ever be found is a moot point. Mental illness cannot be discovered to be caused by a gene or lesion. Tom and I agreed on this point repeatedly. This fact is lost on far too many people. Even if people accepted the fact that mental illness is a contradiction, we are still faced with the activities conducted by institutional psychiatry that are clearly unconstitutional: involuntary commitment, and the insanity defense. The confusion between metaphor and literal disease, brain and mind, is something I believe will eventually be acknowledged by true scientists, jurists, and policymakers. However, those who enjoy the power of depriving innocent persons of liberty, and guilty persons of responsibility, will in my opinion hold on to doing what they believe is right for at least two reasons: (1) They do not want to give up their investments in achieving power. They enjoy having power over other people (2) Society wants to give them this power to put away society's unwanted.

Tom and I frequently discussed what needed to be done in order to strike a mortal blow to the insanity defense and to involuntary commitment procedures. In the former, as he liked to say, a guilty person is regarded as innocent. In the latter, an innocent person is regarded as guilty of a crime. I end here with final discussion regarding this point.

Legal Fiction

When Tom and I argued, I tended to focus on the necessity for exposing mental illness and the insanity defense as legal fiction. A legal fiction, according to *Black's Law Dictionary (4th ed.)*, is:

> An assumption or supposition of law that something which is or may be false is true, or that a state of facts exists which has never really taken place . . . A rule of law which assumes as true, and will not allow to be disproved, something which is false, but not impossible.

As Tom pointed out in his book entitled *Insanity: The Idea and Its Consequences* (1987):

> In the American historical-legal experience, the classic example of a legal fiction is the status of the Negro slave as part-person or property. . . . The idea that some individuals who *seem* to be adult men and women, with appropriate rights and responsibilities are *in law* (de jure)—and hence also *in fact* (de facto)—not really persons because they are insane—is, in my opinion, also a legal fiction.

I told Tom that we must expose insanity and mental illness as legal fiction used to support the insanity defense and involuntary commitment. Tom disagreed. It was hardly the first time he and I argued about something like this. Tom said, "Jeff, we must remove, and prevent, the psychiatrist from being allowed in the courtroom."

I see too many people focusing on how there is no proof that mental illness is a brain disease, as a way of carrying on Tom's heroic work. In my opinion, we should be focused on either of the two issues described immediately above: Exposing the insanity defense and involuntary commitment as legal fiction, and getting psychiatrists out of the court-room. Both are right. And both are critical to the survival of liberty and responsibility in a free society.

Thomas S. Szasz is gone now. For so many people fortunate to have called him a friend and teacher, he lives on in our memories. Szasz considered the fact that he never established a school of analysis or therapy to be one of his greatest accomplishments. I agreed. The goal of therapy or analysis was to help establish autonomy. If he had started a school, it would clearly have turned into a cult.

Toward the end of his life Tom became more curmudgeonly, especially toward me. I wanted him to inform the world that his ideas would not die with him. There are many of us who know and have been teaching his ideas, perhaps as effectively, if not more so, as he did. I wish he had made a point of saying so. He was more than a little difficult in this regard. He was, in my opinion, insecure and competitive. I was fortunate to have taught at least fourteen different college and graduate level courses, using every aspect of his writings in each course, in every book he wrote. My students frequently followed me from one course to the next, and they hungered for more. I remember how one psychology major said to me, "why weren't we ever taught this before?" Too many administrators and faculty members were intent on suppressing Tom's ideas. He was considered "dangerous." He was neither safe nor dangerous, good nor bad.

He was a man, nothing more, nothing less.

References

American Psychiatric Association. (2015). *Diagnostic and statistical manual of mental disorders Volume 5* (5th ed.). Washington, DC: American Psychiatric Association Press.

Black, H. C. (1968). *Black's law dictionary* (rev. 4th ed., p. 751). St. Paul, MN: West.

Schaler, J. A. (1991). Drugs and free will. *Society,* September 28(6).

Schaler, J. (1995). *Introduction of Thomas Szasz as keynote speaker at the Conference for Treaty 6 First Natinos of Alberta. Alternative approaches to addictions and destructive habits.* Edmonton, Canada. http://www.schaler.net/albertaintro.html

Schaler, J. (1999). *Acceptance speech on receiving the Thomas Szasz Award for Outstanding Contributions to the Cause of Civil Liberties.* Washington, DC: Cato Institute. http://www.schaler.net/szaszaward.html.

Schaler, J., Sullum, J., Frances, A., & Pustanik, A. C. (2012). Mental health and the law. http://www.cato-unbound.org/issues/august-2012/mental-health-law

Suzuki, D. T. (1973). *Zen and Japanese culture* (p. 92). Princeton, NJ: Princeton University Press.

Szasz, T. (1963). *Law, liberty and psychiatry: An inquiry into the social uses of mental health practices* (p. 212). Syracuse, NY: Syracuse University Press.

Szasz, T. (1970). *The manufacture of madness: A comparative study of the inquisition and the mental health movement* (p. 179 [footnote]). Syracuse, NY: Syracuse University Press.

Szasz, T. S. (1973). *The second sin* (p. 113). Garden City, NY: Anchor/Doubleday.

Szasz, T. S. (1987). *Insanity: The idea and its consequences.* New York: Wiley.

10

Knoem

Ron Leifer

Now lifeless bone and ash, my friend
To Where has your reason flown?
Now enshrined in immortal print
A different way to think is shown
But why did you choose to not exist
Is oblivion better than life?
Or did you want to escape the strife
That reason brought to your life?
As you know, when you are wrong and society is right
You've made an error
when you are right and society is wrong
you've committed
a heresy
ask Galileo.

About the Authors

BRUCE ALEXANDER, PhD, is professor emeritus of psychology at Simon Fraser University. His two most recent books are *The Globalization of Addiction: A Study in Poverty of the Spirit* (2008) and *A History of Psychology in Western Civilization* (coauthored with Curtis Shelton, 2014). E-mail: alexande@sfu.ca; website: www.brucekalexander.com

MICHAEL SCOTT FONTAINE, PhD, is associate professor of classics and acting dean of the University Faculty at Cornell University. He has published three books on the stage comedy and everyday life of ancient Rome. At the 2014 meeting of the American Psychiatric Association, he spoke "On Religious and Psychiatric Atheism: The Success of Epicurus, the Failure of Thomas Szasz." His website is at http://classics.cornell .edu/people/detail.cfm?netid=mf268. E-mail: mf268@cornell.edu Dr. Fontaine received the Thomas Szasz Award for Outstanding Contributions to the Cause of Civil Liberties in 2016.

RON LEIFER, MD, MA, is a physician trained as a psychiatrist under Thomas Szasz. He received a master's degree in philosophy mentored by the Cambridge philosopher of language and mind, A. R. Louch. Leifer has published five books on psychiatry and Buddhism, some of which can be seen on his website, http://ronleifer.zenfactor.org. E-mail: RonLeifer@aol.com. Dr. Leifer received the Thomas Szasz Award for Outstanding Contributions to the Cause of Civil Liberties in 2001.

HENRY ZVI LOTHANE, MD, DLFAPA, is clinical professor of psychiatry at the Icahn School of Medicine, Mount Sinai, NYC. He has written extensively on the celebrated German Judge Daniel Paul Schreber and plans on writing a book about Sabrina Speilrein. Email: henry@lothane .com Dr. Lothane received the Thomas Szasz Award for Outstanding Contributions to the Cause of Civil Liberties in 2011.

JOANNA MONCRIEFF, MD, is a senior lecturer in psychiatry at University College London and a practicing consultant psychiatrist. She is one of the founders and cochairperson of the Critical Psychiatry Network. She has written *The Bitterest Pills* (2013), *A Straight Talking Introduction to Psychiatric Drugs* (2009), and *The Myth of the Chemical Cure* (2007). E-mail: j.moncrieff@ucl.ac.uk; website: http://joannamoncrieff.com

SUSAN PETRILLI, PhD, Seventh Sebeok Fellow of the Semiotic Society of America, is Professor in Philosophy and Theory of Languages at the University of Bari Aldo Moro, Italy, and Visiting Research Fellow at The University of Adelaide. She has written *The Global World and Its Manifold Faces: Otherness as the Basis of Communication* (2016), *Victoria Welby and the Science of Signs* (2015), *Sign Studies and Semioethics: Communication, Translation, and Values* (2014), and *The Self as a Sign, the World, and the Other* (2013). E-mail: susan.petrilli@gmail.com; website: www.susanpetrilli.com

AUGUSTO PONZIO is professor emeritus and full professor in philosophy and theory of languages at the University of Bari Aldo Moro, Italy. Augusto Ponzio has authored *Lineamenti di semiotica e di filosofia del linguaggio* (2016), *Tra semiotica e letteratura. Introduzione a Bachtin* (2015), (with Susan Petrilli), *Semioetica e comunicazione globale* (2014), *Fuori luogo. L'esorbitante nella riproduzione dell'identico* (2013), and *Il linguaggio e le lingue* (2013). E-mail: augustoponzio@libero.it; website: www.augustoponzio.com

JEFFREY A. SCHALER, PhD, MEd, taught at Johns Hopkins University and full time as a professor at American University's School of Public Affairs. He has edited or authored *Thomas Szasz Under Fire: The Psychiatric Abolitionist faces his Critics* (2004); *Peter Singer Under Fire: The Moral Iconoclast Faces his Critics* (2009), *Howard Gardner Under Fire: The Rebel Psychologist Faces His Critics* (2006), *Addiction Is a Choice* (2000); *Drugs: Should We Legalize, Decriminalize, or Deregulate?* (1998), and *Smoking: Who Has the Right?* (coedited with Magda Schaler-Haynes, 1998). E-mail: Jeffrey@Schaler.net; website: www.schaler.net. Dr. Schaler received the Thomas Szasz Award for Outstanding Contributions to the Cause of Civil Liberties in 1999.

DAVID RAMSAY STEELE, PhD, is the author of *Orwell Your Orwell: A Worldview on the Slab* (2017), *Atheism Explained: From Folly to Philosophy* (2008), and *From Marx to Mises: Post-Capitalist Society and the Challenge of Economic Calculation* (1992), as well as coauthor of *Therapy Breakthrough: Why Some Psychotherapies Work Better than Others* (with Michael R. Edelstein and Richard K. Kujoth, 2013). He is Editorial Director of Open Court Publishing Company, Chicago. E-mail: dramsaysteele@gmail.com

RICHARD E. VATZ, PhD, is professor of political rhetoric and communication at Towson University. He is the author of *The Only Authentic Book of Persuasion* (McGraw-Hill, 2017) and coeditor with Lee S. Weinberg of *Thomas Szasz: Primary Values and Major Contentions* (1983). He has published hundreds of articles, reviews, and blogs. E-mail: rvatz@towson.edu; website: http://pages.towson.edu/vatz/newcv2.htm. Dr. Vatz received the Thomas Szasz Award for Outstanding Contributions to the Cause of Civil Liberties in 1993.

The Thomas S. Szasz Award for Outstanding Contributions to the Cause of Civil Liberties is sponsored by The Center for Independent Thought, http://www.centerforindependentthought.org

A website in honor of the memory of Thomas S. Szasz is maintained as a public service at www.szasz.com

Index

Will → agency 77

g. 101
118

119 addiction
120 "
→ 121

AA 152
137 will

138 cult
140 g 141
149   Scientology of Catholic·

AA-V 160
g 188-189

201